Gail Rae-Garwood

Why a Book of the Blogs?

Those of you who have read ***SlowItCKD 2011*** can skip the blog. It's basically the same information for those who are reading the books in the ***SlowItDownCKD*** series out of order.

When my family doctor told me I probably had a problem and it had to do with my kidneys, maybe Chronic Kidney Disease, my first reaction was to demand in no uncertain terms, "What is it and how did I get it?" Hence, the former title of my blog and the book with which it began.

There are many, many of us out there. By us, I mean those who have Chronic Kidney Disease. Friends, lovers, family of CKD patients can gain some insight into the daily travails of living with the disease via this blog, too. I am no expert, but I have read just about every book concerning this problem that I could find. Of course, most medical texts are not included because I couldn't understand them. Most of the kidney disease cookbooks aren't included because I can understand a heavy duty medical text better than I can a cook-book. I even read memoirs and biographies to glean what information I could.

Surprisingly, very few of these books dealt with the early or moderate stages of the disease. These are the stages when we, as sufferers, are most shocked, con-fused, depressed and at sea. I didn't want to read about transplants or kidney failure. They scared me and I just wasn't ready to learn about them. I'm still not.

But I did want to know what was happening to me on a daily basis, what the medications that were ordered for me were supposed to do, and what new discoveries there were that might help slow down this deterioration of my kidneys. That's what this blog is about.

The more you know about Chronic Kidney Disease and the more anecdotes you read about other people's relationship   with it, the more comfortable you'll feel in the early or moderate stages of having the disease yourself. I sure wish someone had blog-ged about it when it was new to me.

I've discovered I have readers all over the world and they're not afraid to tell me what they need to know. I research for them and respond with a blog post, but remind them they need to speak with their nephrologist and/or renal nutritionist before taking any action.

I did write a first book about Chronic Kidney Disease that you'll find referenced many times in the blogs. That book is **What Is It and How Did I Get It? Early Stage Chronic Kidney Disease**. You can find it in digital on both Amazon.com and B&N.com, as well as in print. **SlowItDownCKD 2011**, originally the first part of **The Book of Blogs: Moderate Kidney Disease, Part 1**, is also available on the same sites.

I started the blog after a doctor in India contacted me telling me he wants his patients to have the first book, but sometimes they can't even afford the bus fare to the clinic. I suggested I start the blog {Not having a clue how to do that}, he translate it, then print it and give it to patients. The idea was that those who could make it to the clinic would bring the printed copies of the blog back to their villages.

Once I exhausted the chapters of the book, I didn't want to stop. This is one of the most rewarding services I've ever performed.

I've omitted the blog posts about websites that no longer exist, products that no longer exist, or services that are no longer available. When you see a set of braces rather than quotation marks, it's me inserting my thoughts into an article.

In the interest of keeping the book from becoming mammoth, I've removed the pictures and a great many references to what was happening at that time in my personal life. I also removed my signature line: "Until next week, keep living your life!" After all, how many times can you read the same sentence in a single book?

When that still didn't shorten the book enough, I removed all notices of past book signings, book talks, Twitter chats, inter views, radio shows, and articles that I'd been involved with. You can't very well go back to the past to attend them, listen to them, or read them from dead links, so why include them I reasoned.

This book was originally the latter half of *The Book of Blogs: Moderate Stage Chronic Kidney Disease, Part*

1. That book proved too unwieldy for comfort. I've used larger type, added a more comprehensive index, and made the book easier to hold since it's only one half the size it originally was.

Enough already! Without further ado, welcome to ***SlowItDownCKD 2012.***

Keep living your life,
Gail

p.s. Bear, you didn't think I'd forget to thank you for accepting
that Monday is reserved for writing the blog, did you?   Many thanks for respecting that, you thoughtful husband, you.

Bedtime is Best

1/2/12   Ladies and Gentlemen, welcome to the first post of 2012. Here's hoping you have the very best year you've had to date.

Dr. Kevin Pho started my New Year right by posting an excerpt from ***What Is It and How Did I Get It? Early Stage Chronic Kidney Disease*** on his blog. I am constantly overwhelmed by the kindness of the medical professionals in helping me with my quest to get the book into the hands of every newly diag-nosed CKD patient.

I've posted about taking cholesterol medication at night and am doing so myself. Then I ran across this article from MedicineNet.com and will explore whether or not to also take hypertension med-ication at night. It all makes sense to me, but I would suggest you talk it over with your nephologist before you make any changes in your med-ication taking regiment.

Blood Pressure Drugs at Bedtime May Cut Heart Risk

Taking at least one blood pressure medicine at bedtime cuts the risk of heart problems, according to new research.

The study also shows that participants taking at least one blood pressure pill at bedtime had lower blood pressure while asleep.

Earlier studies have suggested that bedtime dosing of at least one blood pressure medication may help control blood pressure. But the new study is believed to be the first to look at whether the timing makes a difference in terms of heart attacks, strokes, and death.

Ramon C. Hermida, PhD, director of the bioengineering and chronobiology labs at the University of Vigo in Spain, and studied 661 people with both high blood pressure and Chronic Kidney Disease.

"Taking blood-pressure-lowering medication at bedtime, compared to all medication upon awakening, not only improved blood pressure control, but significantly reduced the risk of cardio-vascular events," Hermida says in a news release.

The research appears in the *The Journal of The American Society of Nephrologists.*

Timing of Blood Pressure Medicines

Hermida's team asked half of the men and women to take all their blood pressure medicine when they got up in the morning. On average, each person took two medicines. Many took more than three. The researchers asked the other half to take at least one of their blood pressure medicines at bedtime.

They measured blood pressure by using 48-hour ambulatory monitoring at the start of the study —

not just a single daytime measurement used in most earlier studies. They also measured blood pressure three months after any treatment changes or, at the least, every year.

The researchers followed the men and women for about five and a half years. They looked to see which heart problems developed. They tracked death from any cause and from heart disease or stroke. They also tracked heart attack, angina, heart failure, and other problems.

More than half of those with Chronic Kidney Disease also have high blood pressure, according to the National Kidney Foundation. High blood pressure increases the risk of the kidney disease worsening. Overall, one in three U.S. adults has high blood pressure, according to the researchers.

Bedtime Dosing of Blood Pressure Medicine

Those who took at least one blood pressure medicine at bedtime had lower nighttime blood pressure while asleep. They were also more likely to have overall good control of their blood pressure. The bedtime group was one-third as likely to have heart and blood vessel problems such as heart attack, stroke, or heart failure, the researchers found.

Improved overnight blood pressure with bedtime dosing had a real benefit. Each 5-point drop in sleep-time blood pressure was linked with a 14%

reduction in risk for heart attack, stroke, or heart failure.

"Cardiovascular event rates in patients with hypertension can be reduced by more than 50% with a zero-cost strategy of administering blood pressure-lowering medications at bedtime rather than in the morning," Hermida says in a news release.

Why Blood Pressure Drugs Work Best at Bedtime

Hermida tells WebMD that some of the body's blood pressure control systems are most active while we sleep. So medicines designed to control those systems work better when taken close to the time when the systems are activated most fully.

The study results "make absolute sense to me," says Robert Graham, MD, MPH, an internist and director of residency research at Lenox Hill Hospital. Graham, an assistant professor of medicine at New York University, reviewed the study findings for WebMD.

"Certain medications have the greatest effect on the body while we sleep," he says. Indeed, bedtime dosing of blood pressure medications recently has been a hot topic among experts. Graham has been prescribing blood pressure medicines to be taken at bedtime for years, he says, as it seems to help with the top side effects of blood pressure medicine: fatigue and drowsiness.

"If you do have high blood pressure, and have
a hard time getting it [down to your] goal,
maybe you should talk with your doctor about
changing the time [you take the medicine]," he says.

EPO Good, No, EPO Bad

1/9/12 In preparing for tonight's Twitter Chat, Libre Clothing {Two delightful young women who started a line of clothing for dialysis wear} asked me about any medications I'd like to mention. I immediately thought of EPO. I remember when I was first diagnosed and complained of fatigue, my nephrologist at the time talked about receiving EPO intravenously. I think he said twice a month.

And I was horrified.I didn't know why; I just was. It wasn't the needle because I was used to that already from all the blood tests CKD patients take and the IVs I'd had for various procedures. It just felt wrong, wrong way down in my gut. Being a great believer in things happening for a reason whether we know the reason or not, I refused. And then I refused again.

After reading the two articles from which I've taken excerpts for today's blog, I'm glad I did.

Blood protein EPO involved in origin and spread of cancer

Researchers at Karolinska Institutet have demonstrated that a growth hormone, PDGF-BB, and the blood protein EPO are involved in the development of cancer tumours and that they combine to help the tumours proliferate in the body. These new preclinical findings offer new potential for inhibiting tumour growth and bypassing problems of resistance that exist with many drugs in current use.

The results are published in the scientific journal *Nature Medicine*.

Angiogenesis is the formation of new blood vessels from pre-existing ones, and is one of the most important research fields in the treatment of such diverse conditions as cancer, metastases, obesity, heart disease, stroke, diabetes and chronic inflammation. The process is also portant in healthy individuals for wound healing, the menstrual cycle and other normal processes. Professor Yihai Cao and his team are researching into angiogenesis and its links to cancer and other diseases, and in the present study show the significant role played by a growth factor, PDGF-BB.

"EPO has several functions," says Professor Yihai Cao. "It produces more blood and stimulates angiogenesis, and we have revealed the underlying mechanism. It also stimulates tumour angiogenesis by directly stimulating the proliferation , migration and growth of endothelial cells and their ability to form the so-called epithelial tube. PDGF-BB promotes the stimulation of extramedullary haematopoiesis, enlargement of the liver and spleen, which increases oxygen perfusion and protection against anaemia."

The introduction of PDGF-BB in mice thus boosts erythopoietin production and the haematopoietic parameters. In addition, EPO may directly act on tumor cells to promote their growth and metastasis. This article is from *Nature Medicine* AOP 4 December 2011.

Then I found a blog written by a doctor as a patient. This is part of that Wednesday, December 07, 2011 blog.

EPO: Lighting the Fires of Cancer
By Peter Laird, MD

Erythropoietin (EPO) is a natural hormone that mediates the production of red blood cells (RBC's) that is primarily produced in the renal cortex and small amounts in the liver. Studies over the last decade evaluated the effects of EPO in diverse populations at risk of anemia outside of the renal dialysis patients, especially in patients undergoing chemotherapy for a variety of cancers.

Unfortunately, these studies revealed adverse survival with more rapidly progressive cancers and shortened survival. In addition, in the CKD population, patients were more likely to experience cardiovascular events and death bringing the CHOIR study to an early close as well.

The TREAT trial followed shortly with a higher risk of stroke for patients treated with EPO for CKD related anemia. Many patients sustained with EPO for years on dialysis vocally protested the new FDA labelling changes and the removal of minimum Hb levels in the QIP. Despite the increased risk of cardiovascular outcomes with EPO and the suspected increased cancer risk for chemo-therapy trials, the correction of anemia for many patients overcame the potential risks.

However, a new study highlighted by Gary Peterson of RenalWEB sheds light on the role of EPO not only in promoting cancer, but it is actually involved in the development of cancers as well:

PDGF-BB modulates hematopoiesis and tumor angiogenesis by inducing erythropoietin production in stromal cells.

As a cancer survivor in addition to my IgA nephro-pathy and dialysis, I have been very leery of EPO right from the time I first started on dialysis in 2007. My first confront ation with my health care team at dialysis came about when I refused to continue EPO shortly after beginning dialysis. In retrospect of current guidelines, I never needed EPO with a Hb over 12.0 with only iron infusions alone.

The issue of adverse cardiovascular outcomes and now this new basic science information that EPO is involved in cancer formation leaves dialysis patients with hard choices. EPO prevents the need for blood transfusions and their associated complications, but at what price?

This is Gail now. For me, this brings up the subject of advocating for yourself. You do NOT need to accept what a doctor tells you or recommends to you just because you are not a doctor and s/he is. Refuse {Unless it's an emergency.} and go home and research...or get a second opinion...or call another patient you trust to suggest another way of finding out if you do need this whatever it is you're not comfortable with.

Getting Back To Basics

1/16/12   I found so many articles that are apt for us that I had a really, really hard time choosing one. I found the winner of that contest at yourkidneys.com.

Learning that you have any disease can be a dis - heartening experience. However, when you are diagnosed with an early stage of Chronic Kidney Disease (CKD) there are many things that you can do to slow its progression, and live a full life. By being conscientious about your health care and lifestyle choices, you can positively affect your quality of life when you have Chronic Kidney Disease.

Tips for living a full life with Chronic Kidney Disease

Here are a few basic tips that may help you slow the progression of Chronic Kidney Disease and live a happier life:
- Knowledge is power – Learn all you can about kidney disease and its treatments.
- Honesty is key – Communicate openly with your health care team and ask the same from them.
- Make lifestyle changes – Be attentive in learning your kidney care plan, take your prescribed medicine, follow the kidney diet and make other recommended changes.
- Think positive – Fill your life with people and things that make you happy. Staying

positive is one of the best choices you can make when you have Chronic Kidney Disease.

Knowledge helps you live a full and happy life
When it comes to Chronic Kidney Disease, there is much to learn, from what type of medicine you need to how you make your diet more kidney-friendly. If you continue to learn all you can about Chronic Kidney Disease, you may feel better equipped to deal with it head on. Ask your health care team any questions you may have.

You can also go online to see if there are local support groups that meet in discussion forums or in person. Communicate honestly with your health care team Your health care team is there to help you manage your Chronic Kidney Disease. It is best to communicate honestly with them so they can best treat the disease.

The kidney diet, medication and other lifestyle tips

Getting answers and guidance to know what to do when you find out you have Chronic Kidney Disease helps you feel more in control of your health. This includes changing your eating habits to include more kidney-friendly foods. To keep your kidneys functioning for as long as possible, it is essential to learn about protein, sodium, phosphorus and potassium, along with knowing how these nutrients make a difference in your health.

Depending on what stage of Chronic Kidney Disease you're in, your renal dietitian will adjust the amounts of protein, sodium, phosphorus and potassium in your diet. In addition, carbohydrates and fats may be controlled based on conditions such as diabetes and cardiovascular disease.

The CKD non-dialysis diet includes calculated amounts of high quality protein. Damaged kidneys have a difficult time getting rid of protein waste products, so cutting back on non-essential protein will put less stress on your kidneys.

Studies confirm that keeping your blood pressure in check can help slow the progression of kidney disease, especially if you have diabetes and/or proteinuria (protein in the urine). According to the National Kidney Foundation (NKF) guidelines, you should keep your blood pressure at or below 130/85 if you have kidney disease, and at or below 125/75 if you also have diabetes and/or proteinuria.

Along with taking your prescribed blood pressure medications, lifestyle changes such as losing weight, exercising, meditating, eating less sodium, drinking less alcohol and quitting smoking can help lower blood pressure. Better blood pressure control helps preserve kidney function.

If you have diabetes, tighter management of your blood glucose level can help slow the progression of kidney disease. It is important to keep your hemoglobin A1C at less than 6.5% or at the level established with your doctor, and closely monitor your blood glucose to avoid hypoglycemia. Ask your doctor or diabetes educator about your diabetes treatment goals and options.

Think positive after your diagnosis

After being diagnosed with an early stage of Chronic Kidney Disease, you are in a good position to take control of your health. Having a positive attitude and surrounding yourself with a support system is necessary to help you live your life to its fullest. As you have learned, there are many ways to slow the progression of kidney disease. Keeping your kidney diet in mind, taking your medicines, controlling any other health issues you may have and changing some lifestyle habits can help. You will have a team of kidney health care professionals on your side to help you every step of the way.

"Fill your life with people and things that make you happy." This sentence popped out at me since that is something I practice. There are fewer people in my life, but these are the people who live on a two way street: one way to them; one way to me.

I almost wish I'd figured this out a long time ago, but then I would have missed out on the fun I had with the others {The ones who no longer want to be with me}, the love that existed then and all the lessons we learned together. I guess it's true that people are in your life as you need them and they need you.

So Tired, Tired of Waiting For…

1/23/12   I'm tired these days with "iron deficiency without anemia" but I clearly remember saying no to Epogen when it was suggested to me in the early days of my CKD. It just struck me as wrong. It was a gut feeling: I knew nothing about it at the time. Since then, it's been suspected of causing cancer and I've written about that in a previous blog.

I've also written in ***What Is It and How Did I Get It? Early Stage Chronic Kidney Disease*** about how it's necessary to remember that your kidneys are not functioning as they should which means that medication may stay in your body longer so you'd need less of it. Has someone heard me? Or was it just time for the medical community to implicate the cautions I'd been suggesting?

On the 19th of this month, EurekAlert.org ran the following.

New drug labels for kidney disease patients — what do they mean?

Drugs that treat anemia are critical for many who have kidney disease

- More than 20 million adults in the United States have Chronic Kidney Disease.
- Drugs that treat red blood cell deficiencies are critical for maintaining many Chronic Kidney Disease patients' health.

- Experts comment on newly released federal recommendations for these drugs.

The U.S. Food and Drug Administration (FDA) recently recommended that clinicians be more conservative when they prescribe Chronic Kidney Disease (CKD) patients with drugs that treat red blood cell deficiencies. But the drug label's recommendations fall short, according to two commentaries appearing in an upcoming issue of the *Clinical Journal of the American Society Nephrology* (CJASN).

The new federal recommendations apply to erythroidpoiesis-stimulating agents (ESAs). Patients with CKD may need these drugs if they lose the ability to make red blood cells and become anemic, which can make them tired, weak, and short of breath. ESAs treat certain types of anemia by stimulating red blood cell production and decreasing the need for blood transfusions. Drugs in the ESA class are epoetin alfa (marketed as Epogen and Procrit) and darbepoetin alfa (marketed as Aranesp).

Clinical trials have shown that ESAs can increase the risk of patients developing heart-related problems such as strokes and heart attacks when used to intentionally increase hemoglobin (a red blood cell component) above 13 g/dL. Because of this, the new ESA label now states that clinicians should consider starting ESA treatment when a CKD patient's hemoglobin is less than 10 g/dL, and they should individualize dosing and use the lowest dose of ESA to reduce patients' need for blood transfusions.

In addition, if a dialysis patient's hemoglobin level approaches or exceeds 11 g/dL (10 g/dL for a CKD patient not on dialysis), clinicians should reduce or hold the dose of ESA. (The drug label previously recommended that ESAs be dosed to achieve and maintain hemoglobin levels within a target range of 10 to 12 g/dL in CKD patients. This target range concept has been removed from the label.)

A commentary by Braden Manns, MD (University of Calgary, in Alberta, Canada) and Marcello Tonelli, MD (University of Alberta, Canada) suggests that the new guidance is not completely consistent with the evidence and that some of the guidance may prove difficult for physicians to apply in practice.

"The recent FDA labeling update seems balanced, although more specific guidance to clinicians would have been helpful," the authors wrote. They suggest that instead of recommending that physicians individualize ESA dosing and reduce it when hemoglobin exceeds 11 g/dL in dialysis patients (10 g/L in non-dialysis CKD patients), perhaps the FDA should simply have recommended targeting hemoglobin ranges of 9 to 11 g/dL in dialysis patients and 9 to 10 g/dL in non- dialysis patients.

In a second commentary, Alan Kliger, MD, Fredric Finkelstein, MD (Hospital of St. Raphael and Yale University), and Steven Fishbane, MD (Hofstra North Shore-LIJ School of Medicine) take a different angle and propose that treatments for anemia should focus on the individual needs of each patient, weighing the risks and benefits in each case. While it is important to minimize patients' chances of developing heart-related problems, it is also important for patients to feel less tired, have more energy and vitality, and be better able to function physically.

"Instead of simply targeting hemoglobin levels, we should be looking at the hemoglobin level in the context of the patients' perception of their quality of life and use ESAs judiciously to improve these perceptions," the authors wrote.

In other words, at what hemoglobin level do anemia-related symptoms become less burdensome for each individual patient? With this information in hand, physicians and patients will be better able to balance the risks versus the benefits of treatment.
You've got to weigh in with your own thoughts on this drug and its dosage. Yes, your doctor is the specialist for your disease, but this is your life. Take charge of it.

Maybe It's Not That Hippy Dippy

1/30/12   I always thought of myself as a wannabe hippy in the '60s. You know, the ones who were attracted to some of the hippy thinking but couldn't quite bring themselves to tune in and drop out or live on a commune. Now, my fiancé and I laugh about the retired lieutenant colonel and the wannabe hippy getting together later in life.

What's even better is that later in my life, the alternative medicine I shocked my parents and colleagues by believing in and practicing is now becoming complementary medicine.I've written about this in ***What Is It and How Did I Get It? Early Stage Chronic Kidney Disease***, but now Catherine Pearson of The Huffington Post has written about it, too.

Nontraditional medical courses like this are be-coming more common and are also offered through many online PhD programs for those with careers looking to incorporate Integrative Medicine into their practices.

How Mainstream Medicine Is Opening Up To Integrative Health

When students elect to spend a month learning about integrative medicine at the University of Maryland, they study by working with the toughest, most frazzled patients: themselves.

In their fourth year of medical school, many of the students are exhausted and fighting to get

good grades. They're tired; they experience head-
aches and back pain; and they don't feel as sharp as
they'd like.

But these students aren't focusing on what drugs to
prescribe. Instead, they're looking at integrative
therapies in search of better health.

Under the direction of Dr. Delia Chiaramonte,
University of Maryland Center for Integrative
Medicine's director of professional education, the
students make a values list, which Chiaramonte says
helps them consider whether they might suffer
from undue stress because they're not focusing
on what's truly important to them. They also learn
to consider how daily stresses and triggers are
affecting their lives, and they practice yoga and tai-
chi.

"By the end of the month, they almost always feel
better themselves," said Chiaramonte. "They really
learn viscerally for themselves that this stuff works."
The Maryland students aren't the only ones looking
past the pill in search of better health. A growing
number of Americans have embraced complementary or intergrative medicine, which combines conventional, allopathic medicine with alternative
therapies.

According to the most recent data from the National
Institute of Health's National Institute for Complementary and Alternative Medicine, some 38 percent
of Americans used some form of alternative
medicine in 2007 — up from 36 percent in 2002.

{This was five years ago! I'll bet that percent is much more than 36 by now.} Experts say such figures explain why a growing number of medical schools have embraced what critics deride as "woo-medicine," but proponents of the techniques say intergrative medicine represents the future of health care.

"More and more students are interested in integrative medicine — that's clear," said Dr. Mary P. Guerrera, a professor of family medicine and director of integrative medicine at the University of Connecticut. "There is greater awareness in the world-at-large. With that, students are coming to medical school already aware of what it is."

In the last decade, the National Consortium of Academic Health Centers for Integrative Medicine, which was formed to promote and support integrative medicine in medical schools, has ballooned from eight member institutions to 51. That list includes top academic names, like Harvard University, Johns Hopkins and the Mayo Clinic.

Last month, University of California-Los Angeles hosted the first-ever National Student Conference on Integrative Medicine, an event created by students looking to build upon the traditional medical school curriculum by exploring topics from what they dubbed an "integrative perspective." It drew more than 100 attendees, including some who don't have access to training in integrative medicine at their home institutions."

I met a resident who wanted to incorporate some of these practices and who said it was so helpful to have physicians who he could talk to. ... It gave him hope that he can go out there and learn this," Guerrera said. "He felt very isolated in his training program, because there was no one he was able to identify to help him."

Among the institutions that do provide training in integrative medicine, that education takes many forms. Some medical schools offer month-long immersive electives, others simply offer several-hour-long lectures introducing medical students to areas they may not have considered before. The University of Arizona has been at the fore-front of incorporating integrative medicine into its programs: They've partnered up with like-minded residency programs and recently created a distinct program for medical students that lets them sup-plement their traditional training with a focus in integrative medicine over their four years.

"It's a really big step that the College Of Medicine was willing to say 'This is important. This is no longer fad, and we will recognize it,' " said Dr. Victoria Maizes, executive director at the Arizona Center for Integrative Medicine.

But some medical schools still lack a formal environ-ment to learn integrative medicine, experts say, and not all institutions have faculty that's supportive of the techniques. That may in part stem from limited evidence testifying to the efficacy of alternative therapies. Even the National Institute for Complementary and Alternative Medicine acknowledges many complementary and alternative medicines lack the backing of trustworthy clinical trials.

But Maizes argued that many tenets of comple-mentary medicine have already been independently verified. She noted, for instance, that there is sig-nificant scientific evidence supporting the role of good nutrition — which is a major focus of integ-rative medicine — in health, as well as the connect-ion between the mind and body. What is lacking, she said, are clinical trials comparing integrative therapies to traditional medicine.

Which is why supporters believe incorporating integrative medicine in medical schools is im-portant, so that students who apply integrative therapies and ideas are well-grounded in convent-ional training.

"We're not cutting anything out from traditional medicine," Chiaramonte said. "We're adding to the toolbox."

It's a Weighty Question

2/6/12 There's a new addition to our family. Little Miss Annabelle is just twelve weeks old and cute as a button, if a kitten can be likened to a button. Thinking about cats led me to wonder if you knew that cats can also have CKD. And if you knew that some of the same treatments are used for feline CKD as for human CKD. That's why you've got to be careful when you do your own research that what you're reading deals with human, not feline, CKD.

This little cutie was introduced to us at a family bar-b-que at which, being human, we overate. That got me to wondering about how hard it's become for me to lose weight, much less maintain a healthy weight. I remembered a blog I'd read on NPR way back in November and decided to share it with you. I can't be the ONLY one concerned with my weight, can I?

Hormones And Metabolism Conspire Against Dieters

There are some fresh insights from Australia that help explain why it's so difficult for dieters to keep off the weight they lose.

Willpower will only take you so far, in case you haven't run that experiment yourself. Turns out our bodies have a fuel gauge, not entirely unlike the gas gauge on our cars, that tell us when it's time to tank up on food.

The gauge relies on hormones that signal to the brain when and how much to eat. But as Dr. Louis Aronne, who directs the comprehensive weight control program at Weill Cornell Medical College in New York, explains, the human fuel gauge can some-imes be way off the mark — especially for dieters.

A study just published in the New England Journal of Medicine documents a pretty extreme diet regimen that limited 50 overweight and obese Australian volunteers to about 550 calories a day for 10 weeks.

Most of them, though not all, actually stuck with the diet, and, not surprisingly, lost a lot of weight. While dieting they shed an average of nearly 30 pounds, or 14 percent of their body weight. At a year, they'd still kept a lot of the weight off, but, on average, their loss was down to 8 percent 15 months after the start of the study.

What happened to their hormones? The researchers measured a whole bunch of them, including insulin, leptin (an appetite suppressant) and ghrelin (a hunger stimulator) and found that more than year after the weight loss, the hormones were telling the people to keep eating — a lot.

As Aronne puts it, their internal gas gauges went down 65 percent instead of the 10 percent or so that would have been more in line with the weight lost. In essence, "they think they're going to run out of gas very, very soon."

So it's not just a lack of willpower that's tripping people up. Their hormones are sending a strong, confounding signal to chow down.

What's more, the study found that the metabolic rate of the dieters remained low a year after the low-calorie diet ended, making it even harder to burn off those calories.

Time for my two cents. While this might be a plausible explanation, I don't find it all that comforting. Yes, I do understand better why I'm having such a hard time with the weight, but I also know this means more exercise to burn off some of those calories my body is holding on to.

So That's What It Means

2/20/12   I have spent almost four years researching, reading, printing, and then promptly forgetting about phosphorous. I keep writing about the three Ps and salt and ending up having to remind myself what phos-phorous is and why we need to limit our intake of it each time I write about it. I was comfortable with pro-tein and easily remembered what I learned about po-tassium, but phosphorous? This one just plain eluded me.

I keep a log of interesting articles I run across just in case there's a Monday that I can't think of anything special. That's what I thought today was going to be. I tried to start the blog with something about the downright beautiful Arabians we saw at the Arabian Horse Show on Saturday and couldn't figure out where to go with that. Then I thought I'd write something about being sick with the flu if you're a CKDer, but worked on that one on the Facebook page. Maybe something about the wood shop being constructed in my garage? Naw. What does that have to do with CKD?

As I was scurrying around making dinner yesterday, my mind consumed with phosphorous, I noticed the bread I was munching on (You know the story: grandfather was a miller in the Ukraine, love of bread in my genes, hardest part of the renal diet for me) tasted salty. Sure enough, when I started poking around in my files, I found this Feb. 7, 2012 article from NPR.com. Notice that last sentence reference to potassium.

To Hold The Salt, It's Time To Hold The Bread
by Eliza Barclay

It's no secret that some of the tastiest snacks around — potato chips, French fries, and processed deli meats — are terrific vehicles for salt. Without salt, they'd be bland, too starchy, or just plain dull.

But would you guess that the white bread on your turkey sandwich could be delivering almost as much as the turkey — up to 400 mg of sodium, or about one-third of the daily recommended limit for 6 of every 10 adults?

A report out today from the U.S. Centers for Disease Control and Prevention unmasks bread and some other sneaky sodium-heavy foods. It turns out that 10 foods — from bread to poultry to cheese to pasta dishes — are responsible for more than 40 percent of people's sodium intake.

According to the CDC, the average American consumes about 3,300 milligrams of sodium per day, not including any salt that may be added during a meal. That's way more than we need, and puts us at risk for high blood pressure, which can lead to heart disease and stroke.

The U.S. Dietary Guidelines recommend no more than 2,300 mg a day, except if you're over 51 years or African American or have high blood pressure, diabetes or chronic kidney disease. For those groups, the recommendation is 1,500 mg a day.

But it's clearly hard to stay within the limits, especially because we can't control the sodium in some of our foods. Some 65 percent of sodium comes from food sold in stores, and 25 percent comes from restaurants. The salt shaker on the kitchen table isn't really the problem — it's the industrial quantities of saline sodium and crystals that are dumped into pro - cessed food to help preserve them and boost their addictiveness.

As public health institutions and other health groups have zeroed in on sodium, sugar and other ingredients in food that can negatively impact health, they're increasingly looking to food companies to make some changes. Some have responded with commit- ments. Kraft Foods, purveyor of such salty snacks as Velveeta and Ritz crackers, said in 2010 it would reduce sodium by 10 percent over a two-year period. Last year, Walmart also said it would cut the sodium in packaged foods by 25 percent by 2016.

Food companies also need to worry about how much potassium is left in food, as Shots has reported. It turns out that consuming a lot of salt in combination with too little potassium is associated with a greater risk of death, according to researchers from the Centers for Disease Control and Prevention, Emory and Harvard.

World Kidney Day Is Only Six Years Old

2/27/12   Each Monday, I find it progressively more difficult to choose a topic. I am amazed at how much information is being disseminated about kidney disease and its treatment and/or underlying causes these days. Since March 8 is the sixth World Kidney Day, I thought we would go back to the basics to start today's blog. Thank you, again and again and again to The National Kidney Foundation for all the information they make available to us. This is their World Kidney Day posting.

Top 10 Reasons to Love Your Kidneys

Sometimes the more you know, the more you love. The National Kidney Foundation urges Americans to get to know two humble, hardworking organs: the kidneys. To help raise awareness and appreciation for all the vital functions the kidneys perform, the National Kidney Foundation offers 10 reasons for Americans to love their kidneys and take steps now to preserve kidney health:

1. Filter 200 liters of blood a day, removing two liters of toxins, wastes and water
2. Regulate the body's water balance
3. Regulate blood pressure by controlling fluid levels and making the hormone that causes blood vessels to constrict
4. Support healthy bones and tissues by producing the active form of vitamin D
5. Produce the hormone that stimulates bone marrow to manufacture red blood cells
6. Keep blood minerals in balance

7. Keep electrolytes in balance
8. Regulate blood acid levels
9. Remove drugs from the blood
10. Retrieve essential nutrients so that the body can reabsorb them

In ***What Is It and How Did I Get It? Early Stage Chronic Kidney Disease***, I discuss how important it is to tell every doctor you see about your Chronic Kidney Disease. Notice #9. "Remove drugs from the blood." You may need to take a lower dosage of whatever drug was prescribed or, perhaps, take it less often. If your kidneys are not fully functioning, the drugs are not effectively being removed from your blood. It would be similar to willfully taking a drug overdose if you do not make your doctors aware of your CKD when they prescribe for you.

Make sure your pharmacist knows about your CKD, too. You cannot rely on your doctors – specialists or not – to remember every warning on every label. That's where your pharmacist comes in. He or she has that same information. You are ultimately the one in charge of your health. It makes perfect sense to draw upon all your resources.

I also discuss in my book the problem in my local hospital's emergency room when I had a bladder infection. Just in case you don't remember, my primary care doctor wasn't available, so her M.A. told me to go to an Urgent Care facility rather than wait since I have CKD. When I arrived and told the receptionist I have CKD, she immediately sent me to the hospital emergency room in case I needed blood or other tests for which the Urgent Care wasn't equipped.

After a battery of tests in the emergency room, sulphur drugs were prescribed, although I'd told them repeatedly about having CKD. Sulphur drugs can harm the kidneys even more.

This got me to thinking about if I were brought into the E.R. under true emergencies conditions – as in unconscious. How would they know I had CKD before they located someone who could tell them about my medical background? Or access my records elsewhere? I knew the answer was a medical alert bracelet, but spent quite a bit of time ignoring the issue. Then I got sick again – a simple flu – but the bracelet idea popped back into my mind full blown, so I started searching for one.

I wanted something that looked like jewelry, but not too much like jewelry because I have simple tastes. So, I did what I do best: researched. I chose a black medical alert plate and had "Chronic Kidney Disease" inscribed on two lines on the back. It's jewelry like, something I'm comfortable wearing and it does the job of making me feel secure should I ever have a true emergency.

Ah, talking about sharing! I found this review of the book on Amazon and walked on air for the rest of the day!

"This is an incredibly well-researched, well-written book written by a woman who herself developed kidney disease. Her book provides clear and comprehensive information for all about the care patients need to have, and responds to the fears and concerns of all involved with coping with kidney disease. It is an honest, very personal accounting of her experience, and I found it to be written clearly, providing tons of pertinent inform-ation about every facet of how to cope with this illness. I think Ms. Rae wrote this book for the ordinary person who learns that they will be living with kidney disease from the moment of diagnosis, on.

But after reading, I believe that it is also a book that every family member, every friend of someone who has develop-ed kidney disease ought to read as well, in order to better understand what their loved ones are going through. I also believe that this book will benefit every professional in the medical community who deals with patients coping with Kidney Disease. It has helped me, and will help everyone involved with the patient on any level to be better able to understand their patient's concerns, anxieties, needs and limitations.

For these reasons I think it is a great guide for the medical community as well as for the patient/family/friends, as it can help professionals understand the kind of information their patients need to have in order to take good care of themselves.

Don't pass this book up!"

National Kidney Month and Doctors Who Get It

3/5/12   Yesterday, day four of National Kidney Month, my buddy and I met at our state theater to see a play I knew nothing about. For me, it was just an excuse to get together. The play, "Dead Man's Cell Phone," turned out to be about what happens to a trafficker in human organs and the people he's connected to after he dies.

What struck me was that I unwittingly chose to attend a play about kidneys during National Kidney Month. At the talk with the actors after the play, I mentioned that. Not one person in the theater {And it was half full of people who stayed for the talk} knew this is National Kidney Month.

We patients are not the only ones trying to be aware. This *New York Times article* can give us some insight into what some of our doctors are doing to stay aware.

Teaching Doctors to Be Mindful

Doctors from across the world gather at the Chapin Mill Retreat Center in Batavia, N.Y., to bring intention, attention and reflection to clinical practice. It was 6:40 in the morning and nearly all of the doctors attending the medical conference had assembled for the first session of the day.

But there were no tables and chairs in sight, no lectern, no run-throughs of PowerPoint presentations. All I could make out in the early morning darkness were the unmoving forms of my colleagues, cross-legged on cushions and raised platforms, eyes closed and hands resting with palms upward in their laps.

They were learning to meditate as part of a mindful communication training conference, held last week at the Chapin Mill Retreat Center in western New York, and sponsored by the University of Rochester Medical Center. There has been a growing awareness among doctors that being mindful, or fully present and atten-tive to the moment, not only improves the way they engage with patients but also mitigates the stresses of clinical practice.

Mounting paperwork demands and other time and productivity pressures can lead to physician burnout, which affects as many as one in three doctors, recent studies have shown. The loss of enthusiasm and engage-ment that results can lead to increased errors, decrea-sed empathy and compasssion toward patients and poor professionalism.

Other problems include physician substance abuse, abandonment of clinical practice and even suicide. Despite the pervasiveness of burnout, few interventions have been shown to be effective.

But two years ago, University of Rochester research-ers studied the effects of a yearlong course for practi-cing primary care physicians in mindful commun-ication. Their findings, published in *The Journal of the American Medical Association*, showed that doctors who took part in the course became more present, attentive and focused on the moment and less emotion ally exhausted over time. Moreover, the doctors' ability to empathize with patients and understand how patients' family and work life or social situation could influence their illness increased and persisted even after the course had ended.

"Mindful communication is one way for practitioners to feel more 'in the game' and to find meaning in their practice," said Dr. Michael S. Krasner, an associate professor of clinical medicine at Rochester and one of the study authors. He, along with his co-author Dr. Ronald Epstein, a professor of family medicine, psychiatry and oncology at Rochester, developed the course in mindfulness.

But it takes training, and that training can be particularly challenging for physicians who are used to denying their personal responses to difficult situations. In addition to learning to meditate, doctors participate in group discussions and writing and listening exercises on topics like medical errors, managing conflict, setting boundaries and self-care. Small group discussions are meant to increase aware-ness of how one's emotions or physical sensations influence behaviors and decisions.

In one exercise, for example, doctors are asked to write about a mistake in their professional or personal life. Examples of such errors have included missing a diagnosis, prescribing the wrong medication, making assumptions about a patient that led to inadequate care or failing to be present for their own families because of an inability to balance work and family life.

The doctors must then discuss the issue with two peers, describing not only the event but also any associated physical and emotional sensations. One of the other doctors has the task of practicing appreciative in-quiry, or listening without making judgments or jumping to conclusions. And the other serves as an observer, offering suggestions at the end of the session for how the listener might improve his or her skills.

Many of the participants at last week's conference, capped by the organizers at 40 and coming from the United States and Canada and from as far away as New Zealand, described the four-day experience as "transformative."

"I can honestly say that these have been some of the most important days of my life," said Dr. Elissa Rubin, a pediatrician and lactation consultant who traveled to the conference from Mineola, N.Y., on Long Island.

But the real challenge for these participants — and the growing number of advocates of such training — is not acquiring mindfulness. It is finding the time and support necessary to sustain their skills and teach others.

Once back in their work environments, many say it is easy to fall back into old patterns. Dr. Krasner and Dr. Epstein have had to close down some of their pro-grams directed at interns and residents because of financial issues. And a frequent topic of conversation among several of last week's participants who hoped to teach at their own institutions were how to best introduce these ideas to colleagues who might be skeptical or administrators who might be hesitant to set aside valuable clinical time for training courses or pay for a program that does not generate revenue.

Nonetheless, Dr. Krasner and Dr. Epstein remain optimistic, in large part because they believe that mindful communication is not just another optional skill or fringe fad in health care.

"Mindfulness," Dr. Epstein said, "and the self-awareness it cultivates, is a fundamental ingredient of excellent care."

Their patients would agree. In clinic, a patient who has suffered for years from chronic pain told me why he remained Dr. Epstein's patient. "He's the best doctor I've ever had because he can get to what I am trying to say quicker than any other doctor. I'm not sure how he does it, but he just really gets it."

World Kidney Day Is Over, But It's Still National Kidney Month

3/12/12 Maybe it's because I'm so enmeshed with anything early stage Chronic Kidney Disease, but I find myself constantly surprised by all the people who don't know a thing about it – many of them suffering from high blood pressure {The second most prevalent cause of CKD} or diabetes {The first most prevalent cause of CKD}. I shouldn't be. I was one of them until I was diagnosed… and that's why I'm so adamant about 'getting the word out there,' as I've come to call my passion.

One of my daughters, Nima – who is a blogger, asked me to guest blog about this issue last week. We talked about it first. I told her I was still angry that, because I have CKD, the chances of her {And her sister} developing it is higher. She asked me questions about the diet and exercise. While she was visiting, we ended up sharing a meal each and every time we went to a restaurant and leaning more toward the food on the renal diet rather than food that isn't. Right now, she's walking my dog while I blog. *Sigh* Guess I'll have to figure out my own exercise for today later.

Maybe today is the day to go back to basics about dealing with Chronic Kidney Disease in my blog. Let's start with the American Kidney Fund's information.

Eat a diet low in salt and fat
Eating healthy can help prevent or control diabetes, high blood pressure and kidney disease. A healthy diet has a balance of fruits, vegetables, whole grains, dairy pro-

ducts, lean meats and beans. Even small changes like limiting salt (sodium) and fat, can make a big difference in your health.

Limit salt
- Do not add salt to your food when cooking or eating. Try cooking with fresh herbs, lemon juice or other spices.
- Choose fresh or frozen vegetables instead of canned vegetables. If you do use canned vegetables, rinse them before eating or cooking with them to remove extra salt.
- Shop for items that say "reduced-sodium" or "low-sodium."
- Avoid processed foods like frozen dinners and lunch meats.
- Limit fast food and salty snacks, like chips, pretzels and salted nuts.

Limit fat
- Choose lean meats or fish. Remove the skin and trim the fat off your meats before you cook them.
- Bake, grill or broil your foods instead of frying them.
- Shop for fat-free and low-fat dairy products, salad dressing and mayonnaise.
- Try olive oil or canola oil instead of vegetable oil.
- Choose egg whites or egg substitute rather than whole eggs.

Choosing healthy foods is a great start, but eating too much of healthy foods can also be a problem. The other part of a healthy diet is portion control (watching how much you eat). To help control your portions, you might:

- Eat slowly and stop eating when you are not hungry anymore. It takes about 20 minutes for your stomach to tell your brain that you are full.
- Check nutrition facts to learn the true serving size of a food. For example, a 20-ounce bottle of soda is really two and a half servings.
- Do not eat directly from the bag or box. Take out one serving and put the box or bag away.
- Avoid eating when watching TV or driving.
- Be mindful of your portions even when you do not have a measuring cup, spoon or scale.

Be physically active
Exercise can help you stay healthy. To get the most benefit, exercise for at least 30 minutes, 5 days of the week. If that seems like too much, start out slow and work your way up. Look for fun activities that you enjoy. Try walking with a friend, dancing, swimming or playing a sport. Adding just a little more activity to your routine can help. Exercise can also help relieve stress, another common cause of high blood pressure.

Keep a healthy weight
Keeping a healthy weight can help you manage your blood sugar, control your blood pressure, and lower your risk for kidney disease. Being overweight puts you more at risk for diabetes and high blood pressure. Talk to your doctor about how much you should weigh.

If you are overweight, losing just a few pounds can make a big difference.

Control your cholesterol
Having high cholesterol, especially if you have diabetes, puts you more at risk for kidney disease, heart disease and stroke. It can also cause diabetic kidney disease to get worse faster. For most people, normal cholesterol levels are:

- Total Cholesterol: Less than 200
- HDL ("good" cholesterol): More than 40
- LDL ("bad" cholesterol): Less than 100

Your triglycerides are also important. People with high triglycerides are more at risk for kidney diisease, heart disease and stroke. For most people, a healthy trigly-ceride level is less than 150. If your total cholesterol, LDL or triglycerides are high, or if your HDL is low, talk to your doctor. Your doctor may suggest exercise, diet changes or medicines to help you get to a healthy cholesterol level.

Take medicines as directed
To help protect your kidneys, take medicines as direct-ed. Some medicines may help you manage conditions that can damage your kidneys, like diabetes or high blood pressure. Ask your doctor how to take any med-icines he or she prescribes. Make sure to take the med-icines just how your doctor tells you. This may mean taking some medicines, like blood pressure medicines, even when you feel fine.

Other medicines can harm your kidneys if you take them too much. For example, even over-the-counter pain medicines can damage your kidneys over time. Follow the label directions for any medicines you take. Share with your doctor a list of all of your medicines (even over-the-counter medicines and vitamins) to help make sure that you are not taking anything that may harm your kidneys.

Limit alcohol
Drinking alcohol in large amounts can cause your blood pressure to rise. Limiting how much alcohol you drink can help you keep a healthy blood pressure. Have no more than two drinks per day if you're a man and no more than one drink per day if you're a woman.

Avoid tobacco
Using tobacco (smoking or chewing) puts you more at risk for high blood pressure, kidney disease and many other health problems. If you already have kidney disease, using tobacco can make it get worse faster. If you use tobacco, quitting can help lower your chances of getting kidney disease or help slow the disease down if you already have it.

Gail Rae-Garwood

Happy Post St. Patrick's Day

3/19/12 I'd forgotten all about my promise to share reviews of **_What Is It and How Did I Get It? Early Stage Chronic Kidney Disease_** with you, so here's another one.

"This is a must read for anyone who has kidney disease. I had the privilege of reading Gail's book and interviewing her on the radio. For anyone with kidney disease, this is one of the best books around written by someone who has kidney disease. I recommend this book highly!!!!!!!!"

Okay, let's get blogging! Now that you've eaten just about everything green you could find, make or buy, it's time to remind yourself of how you should be eating on your renal diet. We all make exceptions in our lives and St. Patrick's Day is a grand excuse to make an exception to the diet. Okay, over, done with, back to the straight and narrow.

I went to The American Kidney Fund's Pair Up site and found some information about the renal diet that I can't accept. While stocking your fridge with already washed and cut fruits and veggies is a good idea, you've got to keep your restrictions in mind – for me it's three servings – each serving size dependent upon the food – of each a day, but also a limited variety. Avoid star fruit!!!! It is toxic to CKDers. Limit the amount of red meat you eat, too.

Or is that just for me? I know my renal diet was adjusted for my likes and dislikes just as yours should be, but I don't know if this red meat restriction is a universal guideline. My renal nutritionist agrees that you needn't cut out your favorite foods, just cut down on them but I think you should cut down on them as a means to cutting them out entirely. Why over-work those poor kidneys? They're already overburden-ed. Whoa! I'm beginning to become the renal diet foodie.

I do agree with everything else in the article and think it's well worth a read.

Living Healthy: Myth vs. Reality

Myth:
It's hard to eat healthy. It takes too much time and doesn't taste good.

Reality:
A few simple changes can make a big difference in your diet.

Some tips:
- Start your day off with breakfast.
- Slow down when you eat.
  - o You may notice that you enjoy your food more.
  - o It takes a while for your stomach to recognize that it's full. Slowing down will give you time to realize you're full before you overeat.
- Stock your fridge with fruits and veggies.
  - o Snack on these instead of chips and crackers.

- o Take time on the weekend to clean and cut them so they're ready to grab and go on busy weekdays.
- Opt for low-fat or fat-free dairy products.
- Switch to whole grain bread and pasta.
- Choose lean meats.
  - o Bake or grill them instead of frying.
  - o Remove the skin from chicken or turkey.
  - o Opt for fresh meats instead of processed meats like lunchmeat and hot dogs.
- Challenge yourself to find healthy recipes.
- Get creative with different combinations of foods and spices.

- Stash your junk food in hard to reach places, like a high cupboard or top shelf of a pantry. When these foods are out of sight and less accessible, you're less likely to indulge.
- Instead of cutting out your favorite foods, limit how much you eat. Rather than eating half a pizza, stop after just one or two slices.
- Avoid eating from large containers. Place one serving in a bowl and put the container away. This can help you keep tabs on your portions.
- Drink plenty of water.
- Eat only when you're hungry.

Gail Rae-Garwood

Popcorn????? Yes, Popcorn.

3/26/12   Well, it looks like that air popcorn maker my children got for me last year is exactly what I need – and I didn't even know it. I thought it was a frivolity, but now it's a health aid!

Before we get to the crunchy stuff, I keep forgetting to post some of the reviews for the book. Doing it first will help me remember.

"Gail Rae's story and book are a terrific resource for anyone facing the challenges of CKD. *What Is It and How Did I Get It?* is an honest, personal, forthcoming account of what it takes to stay on top of your own health. It's great that Gail empowered herself by education and learning — resulting in trusting herself. Hopefully, her story will teach others to take control of their own health by eating the right diet, exercising, and taking the time to understand the myriad of information that comes from the medical world. She does an excellent job of explaining what happens once someone learns they have kidney disease. From what happens with every medical exam, test, visit to a doctor, researching medicines, nutrients, causes, body functions, physiology, etc…touching on every aspect in a very helpful way. This book is a must read for anyone who has any questions about kidney disease, whether it's personal or for a loved one."

Now, air pop some corn kernels, sprinkle powdered cinnamon or garlic or both on it and settle down to read today's article.

Popcorn: The Snack with Even Higher Antioxidants Levels Than Fruits and Vegetables

Popcorn's reputation as a snack food that's actually good for health popped up a few notches today as scientists reported that it contains more of the healthful antioxidant substances called "polyphenols" than fruits and vegetables. They spoke at the 243rd National Meeting & Exposition of the American Chemical Society (ACS), the world's largest scientific society, being held here this week.

Joe Vinson, Ph.D., a pioneer in analyzing healthful components in chocolate, nuts and other common foods, explained that the polyphenols are more concentrated in popcorn, which averages only about 4 percent water, while polyphenols are diluted in the 90 percent water that makes up many fruits and vegetables. In another surprising finding, the researchers dis-covered that the hulls of the popcorn — the part that everyone hates for its tendency to get caught in the teeth — actually has the highest concentration of poly-phenols and fiber.

"Those hulls deserve more respect," said Vinson, who is with the University of Scranton in Pennsylvania. "They are nutritional gold nuggets." The overall findings led Vinson to declare, "Popcorn may be the perfect snack food. It's the only snack that is 100 percent unprocessed whole grain. All other grains are processed and diluted with other ingredients, and although cereals are called "whole grain," this simply means that over 51 percent of the weight of the product is whole grain. One serving of popcorn will provide more than 70 percent of the daily intake of whole grain. The average person only gets about half a serving of whole grains a day, and popcorn could fill that gap in a very pleasant way."

Vinson cautioned, however, that the way people prepare and serve popcorn can quickly put a dent in its healthful image. Cook it in a potful of oil, slather on butter or the fake butter used in many movie theaters, pour on the salt; eat it as "kettle corn" cooked in oil and sugar — and popcorn can become a nutritional nightmare loaded with fat and calories.

"Air-popped popcorn has the lowest number of calories, of course," Vinson said. "Microwave popcorn has twice as many calories as air-popped, and if you pop your own with oil, this has twice as many calories as air-popped popcorn. About 43 percent of microwave popcorn is fat, compared to 28 percent if you pop the corn in oil yourself."

Likewise, Vinson pointed out that popcorn cannot replace fresh fruits and vegetables in a healthy diet. Fruits and vegetables contain vitamins and other nutrients that are critical for good health, but are missing from popcorn. Vinson explained that the same concentration principle applies to dried fruit versus regular fruit, giving dried fruit a polyphenol edge.

Previous studies found low concentrations of free polyphenols in popcorn, but Vinson's team did the first study to calculate total polyphenols in popcorn. The amounts of these antioxidants were much higher than previously believed, he said. The levels of polyphenols rivaled those in nuts {So maybe it's not so bad that we CKDers can't eat nuts.} and were up to 15 times greater than whole-grain tortilla chips. The new study found that the amount of polyphenols found in popcorn was up to 300 mg a serving compared to 114 mg for a serving of sweet corn and 160 mg for all fruits per serving. In addition, one serving of popcorn would provide 13 percent of an average intake of polyphenols a day per person in the U.S. Fruits provide 255 mg per day of polyphenols and vegetables provide 218 mg per day to the average U.S. diet.

National Kidney Month is Over, but You Still Need to Be Aware

4/2/12   All this National Kidney Month activity has only served to make me – and hopefully you – acknowledge how very aware of our kidneys we need to be. I've been in Chattanooga, Tennessee, for an entire week. The Renal Symposium only took one day, but why fly through three time zones for just one day?

I've discovered that I know quite a bit about traveling with early stage CKD. I purposely chose a hotel with an exercise room, but haven't used it once. This is one of those manageable cities so I've walked for miles each day instead. I'm getting older now, so I only walk two or three miles but with all the site seeing I'm barely aware of how much I'm walking.

Most hotel rooms have microwaves and small refrigerators these days, as well as coffee machines. The first day I was here, besides setting up my table for the symposium, I walked 1/2 mile each way to stock up on bottled water, fresh fruit and some vegetables that were already cleaned and cut. My breakfast each day was a cup of my beloved coffee, 15 grapes, half a banana and half a cup of celery. No rushing to get out for breakfast, no ordering food I wasn't comfortable eating and no searching for a restaurant.

What thrills me is that I no longer have to work at knowing what I can eat; it's been long enough that I just know. Menus don't confuse me anymore. If I can't get a child sized portion or one that is senior citizen sized, I can eat as much as I'm permitted to on the renal diet and put the rest in the refrigerator for tomorrow's dinner.

That's another thing. Since the renal diet is so restrictive and I'm already eating actually two thirds of my daily fruit allotment and vegetables at my improvised in-room breakfast, I only eat one full meal out. By the way, that also saves you money you can use for the site seeing and trinkets for the folks back home. I try to eat my protein and starch allotments at this meal since it's so easy to find restaurant meals consisting of this kind of food.

Notice I've still got a fruit and two vegetables left. That allowed me to try a local treat - zucchini with onions baked in cheese with bread crumbs on top. I doubt the cheese was low fat or low sodium, but I used my option to break the diet every once in a great while. Yummy.

I used whatever food units I had left over for late in the evening snacks: animal crackers, ice cream, even a salt-less pretzel. This was the most difficult part of the eating day. It was severely tempting to fall into the I'm-on-vacation-and-I-can-break-the-renal-diet mentality. I did once or twice and was sorry I did. I'm not used to rich cakes or gooey candy anymore and paid for it. That time spent in the bathroom could have been spent seeing more of this surprisingly beautiful city. I didn't expect the headache - and no aspirin permitted, of course - but experiencing this once or twice convinced me all over again that I just wasn't that person who could eat whatever she wanted any more.

You also have to be careful about the bottled water you buy. Dasani adds minerals, the very ones we don't need as CKDers, to theirs. Apparently, they've got the contract for all the local sites here, but I found an acceptable substitute for when I couldn't get any other kind: unsweetened lemonade. I also learned to keep extra bottled water without minerals in my room and take a bottle of it WITH me to the sites so I wasn't stuck with something I couldn't be comfortable drinking.

I've not only learned everything I ever wanted to and more about the Civil War battles and natural wonders of Chattanooga, but also that I'm pretty comfortable traveling with CKD. Here's hoping this week's post has been inspiration for you to get yourself psyched about that vacation you were wondering if you could take.

A Doctor's Advice to Other Doctors

4/9/12   I've had this article from KevinMD.com in my file for months while I decided if it were relevant or not. Obviously, I decided it is.

Why? Because I just had one of these frustrating experiences with one of my own doctors. She raced in, raced out, paid no attention to what I was saying and didn't look at my face once. She is no longer my doctor despite being listed as one of Phoenix's best doctors in Phoenix Magazine's 2012 Top Doctors of The Valley issue.

She IS one of the best doctors here, but I cannot let her just do what she wants with my body when she wants without explaining it to me. Maybe I'm wrong, but one procedure I did allow her to do caused nothing but unnecessary pain without rectifying the condition. And then I discovered she did not give me the proper after care instructions!

I don't think doctors often listen to their patients' suggestions, nor do I think we often give the sugges-tions. We just get angry and change doctors. That is why I was happy to see that Dominic A. Carone, PhD chose to give this advice to her colleagues.

10 ways doctors can lose their patients
As a neuropsychologist, I have the chance to talk to patients throughout the week in detail about their medical histories, supplemented by a comprehensive medical records review. Part of this involves discussing

which provider the patient has seen and if the provider was changed, why. Sometimes, a provider is changed for a benign reason, such as a move or an insurance change but other times there are significant complaints.

Granted, there are always two sides to every story but when I consistently hear the same or similar story from different patients year after year, the stories gain credibility.

Then, when I start to notice the same problems during my own doctor visits, I know there are some serious problems that can be fixed. So, listed below are my top 10 ways for doctors to lose patients from their practice. If you have others to add to the list, please do so.

10. Not accepting lists of symptoms or timelines from patients.

If you see patients, you know they range on a continuum from poor historians who have no idea why they are there to see you and those who arrive with carefully constructed histories that they are eager to give you as soon as you walk in. Just about the worst thing you can do when this happens is to tell the patient that you don't want the list and do not even want to look at it. That connotes a dismissive attitude to the patient and it makes them feel like all of their work was for nothing – work that was done in the hopes it would help you figure out what was wrong. You may have very good reason at the time not to look at the list such as time pressure, but at least take the list and say you will later take a look at it. It will likely provide you some useful information.

9. Asking patients to choose what type of medication they want to take.
When a patient has a medical condition in need of medical treatment, the physician is looked to provide their advice as to what medication to take. They don't want to be given a list of three possible medications, told to research them at home, and come back with a decision. From a patient's perspective, this is why the doctor went to medical school, not me.

8. Long wait times and no apology and/or rushing the patient once coming in.
While no patients want to wait long, they will generally accept the wait time if they are pleased with the care you provide, or if it the initial visit, know that you have a good reputation. However, if the patient waits long and you then walk in and do not acknowledge the wait, explain why there was a wait, and apologize for the wait, it will significantly aggravate the patient. Rush the patient after a long wait and no apology and it will worsen the situation further.

7. Poor bedside manner.
This is an easy one and has been addressed extensively by others, but don't do things such as repeatedly looking at the clock, repeatedly interrupting patients, focusing more on you than the patient, talking rudely, making poor eye contact, etc. Follow the Golden Rule and you will easily establish rapport the majority of the time.

6. Not being responsive to challenging questions.
Provided that a patient is being respectful, there is no reason to become upset when a patient asks

questions challenging a diagnosis or course of treatment. Most patients are generally accepting of your expertise but they may have heard or read something that has given them legitimate questions. Your answers can help reassure the patient that your diagnosis and treatment is correct. Patients are also usually more impressed when you tell them you have no problem with them seeking a second opinion rather than demanding they only accept one point of view and/or becoming overly defensive. Also, patients (or families) sometimes come up with questions that can lead you to entertain an idea you did not previously think of that can improve care. Don't shy away from this. Embrace it.

5. Disrespectful staff.

While the patient may like the care you provide, there are a host of other people they need to interact with before and after the appointment. This includes the receptionist, billing staff, nurses, and others. If these individuals are rude and disrespectful, the patient will likely switch to another provider whose friends and family say have better ancillary staff. It is like owning a restaurant with good food but a terrible hostess and waitress. Many people will just choose a different restaurant. Train your staff to treat your patients the way they would want to be treated (and teach them how to manage patients who are rude) and you will have a happy client base.

4. Drab and dreary office space.

No one likes to go to the doctor. Take some time to make it a more enjoyable experience. Have comfortable seats in the waiting area and waiting room, put some nice art up on the walls (geared towards children if it is a pediatric office), have a TV on with cable (with cartoon options for children), soft music, etc. Whether right or wrong, offices that are bare, uncomfortable, and cold looking convey a message that the patient perspective is not being considered.

3. Being unavailable when needed during routine business hours.
When the answering service repeatedly picks up the phone during normal business hours, it is extremely frustrating for patients. Same with staff not returning phone calls or being absent for 1.5 hours during
lunch time. Patients need to have access to staff during normal office hours to make appointments and ask questions.

2. Cancelling/rescheduling appointments too often. Patients are understanding when a doctor needs to cancel or reschedule but not if it happens too often. This was highlighted in the recent trial of Dr. Conrad Murray, whose former patient testified that after two follow-up appointments were cancelled he felt that the doctor blew him off. The patient never followed up with Dr. Murray again.

1. Making decisions that cause patient harm that were easily avoidable.
While patients will sometimes give doctors a second chance, they won't be inclined to do this if harm occur-red to the patient or a family member that could have easily been avoidable. This is especially true if the harm happened to a child. As a personal slexample, I recall repeatedly explaining to my pediatrician that my child's cough and wheezing was

persistent and affecting her breathing, only to be repeatedly told that it was only allergies, despite the fact that she was cleared by an allergist and was not improving with allergy medications or a nebulizer. Finally, and only by pressuring the phys-ician to do more, was a chest x-ray ordered. Diagnosis: double pneumonia and a week long hospital stay. Totally avoidable. The new pediatrician is very respons-ive and we have been very pleased for many years.

Let's Hear It from the Other Side

4/16/12   A while ago, Dr. Kevin Pho had me guest blog on his KevinMD.com. Recently, I wrote a blog about being in charge of your own treatment. Somehow, somewhere I realized that I'd never advocated for the physician. As a patient advocate, that makes sense; but is it fair? Then I came across this book excerpt on Dr. Pho's site and I had my answer. I had to give the other side the opportunity to be heard.

I need to advise you that I have not read this book, simply the excerpt on Dr. Pho's blog site. However, I do like what the author has to say for the most part. My concern here is if we do attempt to become this friendly and human with the physician, will she {Or he} have the time? It's been clear to me – no matter what kind of doctor I see – that the physician is very carefully watching the amount of time spent with me. Other patients I've spoken with about this have agreed: our beleaguered physicians have only so much time for each patient. I would suggest keeping that in mind as you read the excerpt.

An excerpt from **_The Take-Charge Patient: How You Can Get The Best Medical Care_** _(Lemon Grove Press)which will be released May 15, 2012._

Here are a few suggestions that will help you make the most of your relationship with your doctor. They are for your benefit as a patient, because the more you know, the more empowered you will feel.

Remember That Doctors Are Human Beings

Almost every health care professional emphasized that we all must realize that doctors are people just like us. They have personalities, feelings, good days, bad days, families and social lives.

Sometimes doctors are forced to sacrifice important events to tend to their patients. They miss their kids' soccer games, medical appointments, school meetings and social events. Sure, they chose their profession, but the demands and sacrifices are great. I never realized just how much they sacrifice for their patients until I interviewed the physicians for this book.

Humanize Yourself to Your Doctor

It's easy for us to feel the urgency to get right to the point of why we are seeing the doctor. We begin listing symptoms, talk about how we aren't feeling well, and ask for help. I happen to believe that if we jump right into our symptoms, that is how the doctor will view us— as a set of symptoms she needs to diagnose and treat. I want my doctor to see me as a human being, just as I see her. If she sees me as a human being, then more than likely she will connect to me personally, and that can enhance her willingness to help me. This may not always be possible as some doctors simply are not inter- ested in connecting personally to their patients.

Use Your People Skills

If someone likes you, they are more willing to go the

extra mile for you. This is where your people skills are useful because your doctor will respond to you more positively if you are friendly. That isn't always easy if you aren't feeling well, but I've heard from many doctors that a patient who is angry, bitter, belligerent or has a bad attitude is not well liked.

Being a likeable patient is being a smart patient. Being a smart patient doesn't mean you are faking or being disingenuous. It means you implement strategies to maximize your interaction with the doctor and her staff. You don't have to put up with bad treatment or allow anyone to treat you disrespectfully—I'm not suggesting that you be a doormat. I'm suggesting that being a nice person will get you more of what you want.

Be Nice to Your Doctor

Be nice, polite and appreciative. Many doctors shared experiences with me about patients who were not nice to them. If you aren't nice to your doctor, you are not going to get what you want. Your doctor has something you want that you cannot give to yourself. Do your best to elicit a positive response from your doctor. It's just common sense.

We've all had experiences with doctors who have made us wait forever when we weren't feeling well or whose staff ignored us or were rude or unhelpful. I'm not asking you not to stick up for yourself; I'm asking you to express yourself diplomatically because you need what this doctor has to offer. I try to show goodwill and appreciation toward my doctors not just from a public relations perspective (although that does factor in), but also because I do truly appreciate what my doctors do for me. I am mindful of how far a simple verbal thank you or thank-you note goes.

The goal is to let your doctor know that you value the good care she gives you. If your doctor goes the extra mile for you, express gratitude. We all like to hear that we have done well or that we have done something to improve someone else's life. Doctors need that too. If you complain a lot or approach the doctor and staff with a bad attitude or a sense of entitlement, you are simply not going to get what you want.

If there has been a serious error or act of obvious neglect, channel your anger so you don't come across as out of control. Remember—be firm but respectful. No name-calling or yelling. You only discredit yourself if you yell at doctors and their staff. You look like the villain if you lose control.

Be Nice to the Doctor's Staff

Befriend the doctor's staff. This will help you in a multitude of ways. For example, if you have an urgent message for the doctor, need to see the doctor the same day, need a prescription refill sooner rather than later, or need a procedure scheduled immediately, most of the time you'll get your needs met much sooner if you are friendly and appreciative of the doctor's staff.

Most medical professionals suggested trying to talk with the same person each time you call the office to est-ablish a relationship with that person. This will be your go-to person if you ever have an important need to be addressed. If the front desk person fits you in for an urgent appointment, thank her. This person did you a favor.

Be Nice to the Doctor on Call

Several doctors mentioned the importance of being polite and respectful to the doctor on call—the physician who is covering for your doctor. If you are not, word gets around. This affects how the doctor and her staff perceive you, and it can affect the quality of your medical care.

Act Involved in Your Health

Who knows your body better than you do? You are the expert on you—share with your doctor what you know so she can do her job. Most doctors said that patients who are involved and invested in their health cause them to be more involved and invested in the patient's health. Many physicians said that if a patient doesn't care, it makes their job much more difficult. Many said that patients who don't care aren't going to follow their instructions to get better.

If you think about it, what is your doctor's motivation to go out of her way for you if you give the impression you don't care about your health and medical care? This seems like simple common sense to me, but when you get sick, sometimes that just goes right out the window. I'm not proud of it, but I clearly remember leaving screaming messages on a former nephrologist's answering machine when he would not call me back about surgery I was having in just two days. {I finally had the surgeon call him.} Yes, he was an incredibly arrogant person who had no respect for me, but did it help that I treated him – shall we say – less than respectfully, too? Answer: Nope, it just helped my self-respect fly out the window.

Down In the Mouth

4/23/12 Last Friday, I had an emergency root canal. That was unfortunate {Still VERY tender} for me, but fortunate for you. Why? Well, I'd never even thought about what impact Chronic Kidney Disease might have on dental treatment before. I've learned a little bit and I want to share it with you.

When my dentist poked the tooth and I said, "Don't," he arranged for this root canal the very next day telling me I must see an endodontist. When I met him, we talked a bit about how our disease impacts endodontistry and figured out that the anesthetic is what we needed to focus on. This endodontist not only explained {As I will in a paragraph or so}, but showed me the medical tome he based his decision upon and then lent the book to me so I could quote directly from it for this blog.

The book - which I didn't know even existed - is ***Dental Management of the Medically Comprised Patient, Fifth Edition*** by James W. Little, Donald A. Falace, Craig S. Miller and Nelson L. Rhodus. You need to realize that as CKDers, WE are medically compromised patients. Don't ever forget that.

In a previous blog, I've mentioned my brush with emergency room physicians when I had an as yet undiagnosed bladder infection and they insisted I could take sulphur drugs. They were wrong. I have Chronic Kidney Disease and cannot take sulphur drugs. I didn't want to take the wrong medication again.

As it turned out, the tooth was caught before it became infected so I didn't need any antibiotics, but there was the anesthetic as already mentioned. I was nervous. What would he want to use? Would he suggest I not use any since I was being so insistent that the drug not leave the body via the kidneys? I remembered the pain of a previous root canal over a decade ago. It was so awful that I cringed just thinking about it.

I thought maybe I'd just let him take charge, but couldn't do that. There's a reason I keep telling you to be in charge of your own body. I couldn't abdicate that responsibility because I was frightened. It was just fear of pain.

You see, my mouth is my weak spot since I opened a car door into it when I was 19. Surely, I could figure this out with the endodontist's help so I wouldn't have to endure pain. Remember I don't track very well when I'm scared. That is, after all, the reason I wrote **What Is It and How Did I Get It? Early Stage Chronic Kidney Disease** in the first place.

He gave me the information I asked for and explained it to me as I sat there dumbly. Then I barraged him with questions about what he'd said concerning liver exiting and kidney exiting drugs. Okay, I got it that there was no anesthetic he could use that would exit solely via the liver. Then he mentioned one that only 2% of exits via the kidneys. I am stage three. I was willing to chance that one.

When I finally understood the name he was telling me,

I felt a little foolish {Don't you! You need to question about drugs and treatment.} It was lidocaine. Perhaps you know it as Xylocaine. Either way, it is one of the most common drugs used in such procedures.

Right there, in *Table 11-2 Drug Therapy in Chronic Renal Disease* on page 270, I read that the normal dosage is "okay" and that most of the drug would be exiting via the liver. With my mind at ease, I only felt the initial injection and one quick pain in an area which hadn't been anesthetized enough. The endodontist soon remedied that situation.

I am astounded at how very painless the procedure was… and gratified I was able to take a drug that wouldn't further comprise my already compromised kidney function. I am also thankful for the education and the ease of the process. How nice to know there's
one less thing for me to fear in this world.

So now my lesson is yours. I get such a kick out of personally learning something that I can pass on to you.

Gail Rae-Garwood

As I Sneeze My Way Through Life

4/30/12   Ever since I was a teenager, I've been allergic to cats. For some reason, it got worse when I moved out to Arizona a decade ago. But, wait, what was this? Certain kinds of dogs made me sneeze, too. Luckily, not my sweet Bella who is part Australian Cattle Dog and part German Short-Haired Pointer.

I was becoming uncomfortable and going back to the sneezing and need for lots of tissues without a cat in the house and with a dog who didn't cause these symptoms. What made it even worse is that I love fresh air and would keep the doors and windows open until it hit 90 degrees each day.

It was easy enough to figure out these were allergies, but I thought because I had Chronic Kidney Disease that I couldn't do anything about it. When my primary care doctor suggested they were keeping me up at night - which meant I wasn't getting the eight hours of sleep a night CKDers need, she suggested I see an allergist to see what, if anything, could be done to alleviate the situation.

It turned out that I am not only allergic to cats and certain breeds of dogs, but I now have allergies to weeds and plants that don't live back East. I had been exposing myself to vast amounts of pollen from Firebush, Kochia, Mesquite {Ack! I planted one outside my office window when I bought this house}, juniper, white mulberry and the list goes on and on.

74

I could have simply sealed myself in my house with its no-air-gets-through windows and arcadia doors, but that wouldn't have worked. I need open windows. I need open doors. To me, they are as essential as food.

My allergist carefully explained to me that we could start a regimen of injections but it would take a long time to build up the antibodies. I didn't really care about that since I was getting sort of tired of red eyes and always having a tissue clutched in my hand. I was concerned about what was in those injections.

Once she explained, I had one of those why-didn't-I-consider-this years ago moments. They contained minute portions of each of the substances I was allergic to. There were no chemicals in them to exit via the kidneys. In other words, they were safe for a CKDer like me.

According to the American Academy of Allery, Asthma, and Immunology, this is how immunology works. Allergy shots work like a vaccine. Your body responds to the injected amounts of a particular allergen (given in gradually increasing doses) little by little, developing a resistance and tolerance to it. Allergy shots can lead to decreased, minimal or no allergy symptoms when you are again exposed to the allergen(s) in the shot.

You ARE Part of the Process

5/7/12   The article I've included today has to do with the idea that the patient must have a say in determining which tests {s}he takes and is written from a physician's point of view. I discuss this in **What Is It and How Did I Get It? Early Stage Chronic Kidney Disease** and you'll notice that some of the reviews mention it, too. This is your body, your life. Certainly you should seek the advice of medical experts, but the decision whether or not to take (insert name of medical test) is ultimately yours.

This post is from KevinMD.com.

Shannon Brownlee's recent post, "Don't discard shared decision making on the basis of PSA testing," couldn't ring more true. The crux of shared decision making is that the patient must decide, with his or her physician, which tests or procedures make sense, given the various risks, tradeoffs and outcomes. Discarding the construct on the basis of one test (PSA testing) is not only poor form in that it is a sample of one, but also what might not seem like much of a choice to some may be the biggest choice of all to someone else.

Choice is the operative word in this debate. Patients need to know their options, regardless of physician opinion or what research says would probably happen (i.e. a false positive). It is up to the patient to choose whether the odds are worth it to them. And while PSA testing may not be strong in validity (though the research does conflict), causing some doctors to (erroneously, in my opinion) consider it non-elective, there are certainly common medical tests that warrant shared decision making, such as colon cancer screening, for example.

In addition to the decision of whether or not to be tested there are several choices about how to get tested and then after that several choices about what to do in the event that a polyp is found. When medical evidence supports more than one approach to testing, patients should be informed about their choices and providers should respect their preferences.

Shared decision making is not just the right thing to do, it is one of the most effective ways to combat the myriad health issues affecting us today – quality, cost, satisfaction. Shared decision making is not meant to encourage or discourage certain tests or procedures – it is meant to involve and educate each patient so that no medical choice is made without them. And that makes patients happy – exercising the right to be involved in decisions about their care.

Once educated, patients do tend to select less invasive procedures on average, as Shannon notes, and costs thereby go down as does the risk of medical error or unwanted care. A randomized controlled trial in the *New England Journal of Medicine* also produced these effects: a shared decision making intervention produced 9.8% fewer inpatient and outpatient surgeries and 11.5% fewer hospital admissions.

Shared decision making makes healthcare better. To my fellow physicians trying to determine whether to test or not to test – include the patient first. Is the patient involved? That is the real first question.

After thinking about what you read above, read the reviews about *What Is It and How Did I Get It? Early Stage Chronic Kidney Disease* below and then get involved in your own life. Ask questions, weigh the options and let your medical expert help you make YOUR decision.

"This book includes TONS of definitions and images and is a good read for anyone looking to learn more about kidney disease — whether you're a doctor or a recently diagnosed patient. Her perspective is real and her stories will relate with many. The book touches on many topics from related health complications to dealing with nephrologists and maintaining a kidney friendly diet.

If you or someone you know is facing CKD, I highly recommend reading this book. Take experiences from those who have already gone through it and are looking to help."

"Gail Rae's story and book are a terrific resource for anyone facing the challenges of CKD. *What Is It and How Did I Get It?* is an honest, personal, forthcoming account of what it takes to stay on top of your own health. It's great that Gail empowered herself by education and learning — resulting in trusting herself Hopefully, her story will teach others to take control of their own health by eating the right diet, exercising, and taking the time to understand the myriad of information that comes from the medical world.

She does an excellent job of explaining what happens once someone learns they have kidney disease. From what happens with every medical exam, test, visit to a doctor, researching medicines, nutrients, causes, body functions, physiology, etc...touching on every aspect in a very helpful way.

This book is a must read for anyone who has any quest-ions about kidney disease, whether it's personal or for a loved one."

"This is a must read for anyone who has kidney disease. I had the privilege of reading Gail's book and inter-viewing her on the radio. For anyone with kidney disease, this is one of the best books around written by someone who has kidney disease. I recommend this book highly!!!!!!!"

"Gail Rae's book, **What Is it and How Did I Get it? Early Chronic Kidney Disease** provides information about this disease from the patient's viewpoint. Having dealt with many doctors while dealing with a different health issue, I have learned how important it is to understand what all the tests and procedures mean. From my viewpoint, it's also important to know how to talk with your doctor and even more importantly in my opinion to know how to get the doctor to talk with you about prognosis, treatments, and any questions you have.

Her book gives you the basic understanding about Chronic Kidney Disease and addresses issues that can puzzle and frighten patients. She gives you her experience as a patient as well as information she's researched trying to find her own answers. A useful resource for anyone dealing with Chronic Kidney Disease."

"This book is wonderful because it explains all you need to know for early stages of CKD and not in medical terms, but in terms that everyone can understand. The author was so passionate about getting the information to others who are going through what she went through as this information was not available to her. Her altruistic motive for this book is also what makes it wonderful. I would definitely buy a copy if I were you."

"Having lived with autoimmune diseases since my late 20's, and I know firsthand what it's like to get a new diagnosis. Even with the internet, it's hard to get solid, reliable and empathic information. This book does it all in an easy to read format. I think this is useful for a person with any new diagnosis be cause it highlights the issues people wonder and worry about."

"As the daughter of a mother who has early stage CKD, I have to admit at first I panicked at the diagnosis. What exactly did it mean? I was relieved to find this book and even more so relieved to find that it was written in plain English and not Medicalese. Author Gail Rae has written an easy to follow book not just for the newly diagnosed early stage CKD patient, but, also for their family members and friends. There's even an entire chapter dedicated to questions raised by friends and family. I highly recommend this book for both the newly diagnosed early CKD AND their family/friends."

"This is an incredibly well-researched, well-written book written by a woman who herself developed kidney disease. Her book provides clear and comprehensive information for all about the care patients need to have, and responds to the fears and concerns of all involved with coping with kidney disease. It is an honest, very personal accounting of her experience, and I found it to be written clearly, providing tons of pertinent information about every facet of how to cope with this illness."

"I think Ms. Rae wrote this book for the ordinary person who learns that they will be living with kidney disease from the moment of diagnosis, on. But after reading, I believe that it is also a book that every family member, every friend of someone who has developed kidney disease ought to read as well, in order to better understand what their loved ones are going through. I also believe that this book will benefit every professional in the medical community who deals with patients coping with Kidney Disease.

It has helped me, and will help everyone involved with the patient on any level to be better able to understand their patient's concerns, anxieties, needs and limitations. For these reasons I think it is a great guide for the medical community as well as for the patient/family/friends, as it can help professionals understand the kind of information their patients need to have in order to take good care of themselves. Don't pass this book up!"

"This book is especially good for the newly diagnosed with CKD. So much information in a well written format. The author, a teacher and a writer uses her excellent skills to make this disease easier to understand and "navigate". Highly recommended. Medical specialists should give this to all of their kidney disease patients."

Thanks for the chance to let you know how others view the book.

Validation That It Is the Most Important Meal of the Day

5/14/12 I'm laughing out loud right now {Remember LOL?}. No sooner did I include the book's Amazon reviews in the last blog than I started getting requests for the Barnes and Noble reviews. Amazing how people seem to root for one bookstore or the other, almost as if they were football teams. So, to be fair, here they are:

"Well written and very informative! This book includes tons of definitions and images and would be helpful for anyone looking to learn more about kidney disease. Gail's perspective is real (even funny at points) and I think anyone dealing with CKD will definitely be able to relate with her stories. This book is beneficial for anyone going through CKD, caregivers, and medical profession-als."

"This book gives great insight and an in-depth look into CKD. What to expect, what to look for, not just as a patient but for those that are in the patient's life as well. Diet, exercise, nutrition, supplements, etc. is all touched on in this book. If you are a newly diagnosed CKD patient, already a CKD patient, or a family/friend of a CKD patient...you will want this book to give you a better piece {sic} of mind of what you're dealing with and how to make your life a little easier at the same time."

"Her blog is also a great resource to use daily too. I wish I had known about this book when my mom was going through CKD before her transplant, it would have helped us better understand everything that was happening, was going to happen, and terminology that the doctors used. A must read!"

"This is an incredibly well-researched, well-written book written by a woman who herself developed kidney disease. Her book provides clear and comprehensive information for all about the care patients need to have, and responds to the fears and concerns of all involved with coping with kidney disease. It is an honest, very personal accounting of her experience, and I found it to be written clearly, providing tons of pertinent information about every facet of how to cope with this illness."

"IF you have recently been diagnosed with Chronic Kidney Disease this book should be your next purchase. Gail Rae shares her personal experiences with the disease, lists of foods which have become part of her diet, how to decipher your medical records, questions to ask your doctors, and what she has learned about living with CKD."

Naturally, reviews are not the purpose of this blog. Let's talk about breakfast, instead. You know Mom always used to say {Well, my mom didn't but the ads on Saturday morning cartoons did}, "Breakfast is the most important meal of the day." And you know, diabetes is one of the two - the other is high blood pressure - most common causes of Chronic Kidney Disease. Here's some information that ties breakfast and Type 2 diabetes together.

Really? To Lower Your Risk of Diabetes, Eat Breakfast

THE FACTS

The benefits of eating a solid breakfast are hard to dispute. People who skip that all-important first meal of the day, studies show, suffer setbacks in mood, memory and energy levels. They are also more likely to gain weight, in part because of excess eating later in the day. Research on the habits of people taking part in the National Weight Control Registry, a long-running study of successful dieters, for example, shows that about 80 percent eat breakfast daily.

But emerging research suggests another advantage to consistently eating breakfast: a reduced risk of Type 2 diabetes. In a study published in the current issue of *The American Journal of Clinical Nutrition*, researchers followed 29,000 men for 16 years, tracking their diets, exercise, disease rates and other markers of health. About 2,000 of the men developed Type 2 diabetes over the course of the study. Those who regularly skipped breakfast had a 21 percent higher risk of developing diabetes than those who did not. The heightened risk remained even after the researchers accounted for body mass index and the quality of the subjects' breakfasts.

Other studies have also found a link between skipping breakfast and greater risk of Type 2 diabetes. While it is not clear why the relationship exists, some scientists suspect that a morning meal helps stabilize blood sugar through the day. Some studies show that consuming a larger proportion of your calories later in the day, especially carbohydrates, has a detrimental impact on blood sugar and insulin levels.

THE BOTTOM LINE

Regularly skipping breakfast may raise the risk of Type 2 diabetes.

Clearing My Head

5/21/12 Today's the day to bring up those isolated thoughts roaming through my mind. I pulled up this article from last Halloween (Hmmm, is the date relevant?) as an example of why I have so many doubts about drugs, drug companies, and just what each drug can do despite the fact that we sometimes need the drug. As for all those questions about Vytorin, this may help.

Controversial Cholesterol Pill Vytorin Shows Promise for Kidney Patients

{The first part of the article refers to a television advertisement demonstrating that your high cholesterol may be caused by genetics, bad habits or a combination of both.}

Remember Grandpa Frank? Way back in 2008, the ad above ran in heavy rotation on TV during the heyday of Vytorin, a cholesterol-lowering pill that claimed to fight both genetics and bad habits.Soon after the ad had appeared, oh, say thousands of times across the country, the Food and Drug Administration asked the company to revise the ads with Grandpa Frank and other relatives because the ads didn't reveal a study showing Vytorin wasn't any more effective than simvastatin, a generic cholesterol medicine that is one of Vytorin's components.

Later that year there was more bad news for Vytorin — and fear among patients — when a study suggested

Vytorin raises the risk of cancer slightly. Sales fell from a peak of $5 billion a year to $2 billion last year. None of this caused the FDA to change its view of the safety of Vytorin. The agency even issued a statement in 2009 essentially exonerating Vytorin of the cancer risk.

Now, Merck, the maker of Vytorin, is looking to regain some of the lost sales of the drug by touting its use in people with Chronic Kidney Disease. A new FDA analysis shows Vytorin lowered the relative risk of heart attacks and strokes by 22 percent among CKD patients in the relatively early stages of disease — before they need dialysis. For those with more severe, later-stage disease, the drop was 6 percent. The FDA analysis also failed to find any increase in cancer or cancer deaths in the 20,000-plus patient study.

Merck is seeking FDA approval for use of Vytorin in CKD patients of which there are 26 million in the U.S. alone, according to the National Kidney Foundation. A committee of independent advisers to the FDA will go over the data for and against Vytorin at a meeting Wednesday.

I've got more questions:

1. Why is Vytorin, rather than its generic form — simvastatin — being touted? Didn't the article state that this component of Vytorin was just as effective?

2. What happened to the study suggesting that Vytorin raises the risk of cancer slightly?

3. Why isn't it mentioned in the article? "In patients with Chronic Kidney Disease and estimated glomerular filtration rate <60 mL/min/1.73 m2, the dose of Vytorin is 10/20 mg/day in the evening. In such patients, higher doses should be used with caution and close monitoring."

4. Where is there mention of further studies discussed in the FDA's report: "With all the controversy surrounding ezetimibe in the past 18 months, the cardiology community anticipates the results of IMPROVE-IT, the large clinical-outcomes study chaired by Dr. Eugene Braunwald of the TIMI Study Group and cochaired by Dr. Robert Califf (Duke Clinical Research Institute, Durham, NC). The study will compare simvastatin 40 mg plus ezetimibe 10 mg with simvastatin 40 mg alone in 18 000 patients with a recent acute coronary syndrome. Those results will be available in 2012.

I do not mean to attack this particular drug from this particular company, but am using this article as an example of just how unsure I am about what we are being told about the drugs we use and how contradictory the information about these drugs can be.

Lest We Forget

5/28/12   Ready for some kidney news? First, do you remember my disappointment with the medical jewelry company that sent the alert bracelet with a note saying that it should not be immersed in water, as in bathing or swimming? I don't know about you, but I have this habit of showering every day and that includes immersing myself in water.

I also have artritis which means taking jewelry off and then putting it back on is a nightmare – even with the arthritis helper made specifically for this purpose. My mother loved that little device; I'm just not coordinated enough with my left hand to use it on a bracelet worn on my right hand since I'm right handed. We can now bypass the whole problem. Read on.

Tattoos Replace Bracelets for Medical Alerts

As more people with diabetes replace their medical alert Ts with tattooed warnings, there might be a need for a standard design and body location, a researcher here said.

"The tattoo has to be easily recognizable to first responders," Saleh Al-dasouqi, MD, from the Sparrow Diabetes Center of Michigan State University in East Lansing, said during a press conference. "It may be that we need guidelines for medical alert tattoos for both patients and tattoo artists," Aldasouqi said. "Should tattoos be prescriptive? I don't know. We're at the beginning of this dialogue and I think it's an important one."

Medical alert tattoos for diabetes are a relatively new phenomenon and Aldasouqi admitted he has no hard data on the number of people who choose ink over metal to alert first responders in case of an emergency. He initially became aware of medical tattoos about 3 years ago when a patient showed up with one. His search of the literature, however, produced only two case reports. But a search on the Internet revealed ample evidence that the practice is alive and well. "You can find groups of people discussing their medical tattoos," he said.

Rick Lopez, who works at Hard Ink Tattoo in Philadelphia, told *Medpage Today* that he recently inked a diabetes alert on a young man. "He brought the bracelet into the shop and I just copied it onto his wrist," Lopez said. He said he has tattooed a lot of "cancer ribbons" on customers, generally family members of those with cancer who want to show support, but also on cancer survivors as well. And he has inked the autism puzzle ribbon. But only one medical alert.

Aldasouqi and colleagues reported a case presentation here of a 32-year-old women with type 1 diabetes who decided to shed the alert jewelry for a permanent ink reminder on her wrist. She said she was frustrated with the numerous broken necklaces and bracelets throughout her life, and the ensuing costs of them.

Last year in the *American Family Physician* journal, Aldasouqi published another case report of a man who tattooed his diabetic condition onto his wrist.

As the practice of medical tattoos grows, he wants to ensure it's headed in the right direction. Paramedics have to be educated about these tattoos so they recognize them during an emergency. There perhaps should be some standardization in design and location, such as the wrist, so it's easier to identify the tattoo as an alert, he said.

He cited a case where a man had the letters "DNR" inked on his chest. During an emergency, first responders thought the tattoo might be a directive for "do not resuscitate." As it turned out, the man had lost a bet in his youth, which resulted in those letters emblazoned on his chest.

Aldasouqi has recently teamed up with a colleague from the University of Helsinki to produce peer-reviewed studies on the phenomenon and to begin a registry of patients with medical tattoos.

The Thing You Don't Want to Talk About

6/4/12 So, what is it you never want to talk about? Your colonoscopy, of course. This is something readers have asked about and it's time to deal with it, unsavory thought or not. If this is a new word for you, once you read WebMD's description, you will realize why no one ever wants to talk about this.

Colonoscopy is a test that allows your doctor to look at the inner lining of your large intestine (rectum and colon). He or she uses a thin, flexible tube called a colonoscope to look at the colon. A colonoscopy helps find ulcers, colon polyps, tumors, and areas of inflammation or bleeding.

During a colonoscopy, tissue samples can be collected (biopsy) and abnormal growths can be taken out. Colonoscopy can also be used as a screening test to check for cancer or precancerous growths in the colon or rectum (polyps).

The colonoscope is a thin, flexible tube that ranges from 48 in. (122 cm) to 72 in. (183 cm) long. A small video camera is attached to the colonoscope so that your doctor can take pictures or video of the large intestine (colon). The colonoscope can be used to look at the whole colon and the lower part of the small intest-ine. A test called sigmoidoscopy shows only the rectum and the lower part of the colon.

Before this test, you will need to clean out your colon (colon prep). Colon prep takes 1 to 2 days, depending on which type of prep your doctor recommends. Some preps may be taken the evening before the test. For many people, the prep for a colonoscopy is more trying than the actual test. Plan to stay home during your prep time since you will need to use the bathroom often. The colon prep causes loose, frequent stools and diarrhea so that your colon will be empty for the test. {Delightful prospect isn't it?}

The colon prep may be uncomfortable and you may feel hungry on the clear liquid diet. If you need to drink a special solution as part of your prep, be sure to have clear fruit juices or soft drinks to drink after the prep because the solution tastes salty. {You have CKD; this is not the prep you will be using.} The National Digestive Diseases Information Clearinghouse (NDDIC) at The National Institutes of Health (NIH) says this about when to start being tested:

Routine colonoscopy to look for early signs of cancer should begin at age 50 for most people — {Don't you just love these gifts that come with getting older?} earlier if there is a family history of colorectal cancer, a personal history of inflammatory bowel disease, or other risk factors. The doctor can advise patients about how often to get a colonoscopy.

Their material about colonoscopy is well worth looking at, but you need to remember you have CKD and so, cannot take certain substances in preparation for your colonoscopy. You cannot take the usually prescribed Fleet enemas or anything with oral sodium phosphate. Get it? Sodium? Phosphate?

One possible alternative is a polyethylene glycol {PEG} solution such as Miralax and {I think} Ducolax. As usual, check with your nephrologist.

During my own colonoscopy last year {Yay! I'm home free for nine more years since it's suggested the test be performed every ten years}, several polyps were removed; some because they were bleeding, some because they were the larger kind that could become cancerous {adenoma}. Apparently, bleeding polyps are troublesome because they can be the source of your fatigue if you already have low levels of iron as most CKDers do. At least, that's what my nephrologist said, but I'm still tired {Sleep study coming up next month}.

More often than not, you are anesthetized before the procedure, both to insure you do not move which might cause a perforation and for your own comfort. You are a medically compromised patient. I'll repeat that – you are a medically compromised patient. As such, you need to be treated differently as far as anesthesia. I have to admit that the research I found was far too med ical for me. BUT two things were very clear:

1.The dosage of the anesthesia may have to be
   changed and

2. You must let your doctor know on your first visit
   that you have Chronic Kidney Disease.

I was both disgusted and fascinated by the photos my gastroenterologist sent me after the procedure. I saw the polyps. I saw the inside of my colon.

Let's Sleep On It

6/11/12 I've been reading quite a bit about the importance of sleep with Chronic Kidney Disease. In addition, one of the first things my nephrologist mentioned
– after hearing my schedule – when he discussed lifestyle changes was the importance of a minimum of
eight hours of sleep per night.

If I'm crowded {You should have seen the hallways,
the living room and the family room overflowing not
only with books, but book cases.}, worried that the 115
degree heat here is making my house paint chalk
{Which allows more heat in than normal} or wist-
fully thinking about the screened in porch I was no
longer comfortable using {Due to heat? CKD? Age?}, I
am not going to get a good night's sleep. By the way,
that porch is now the library.

These articles will make clear just how important that is.
Keep in mind that you are already at higher risk for having a stroke simply because you have CKD. Add diabetes
and/or hypertension and that risk is heightened.

The first is from USAToday.

Lack of sleep increases stroke risk

The 30% of working adults who routinely sleep less
than six hours a night are four times more likely to
suffer a stroke, says a new study. The findings are the
first to link insufficient sleep to stroke; they're also

the first to apply even to adults who keep off extra pounds and have no other risk factors for stroke, says Megan Ruiter, lead author of the report....

"People know how important diet and exercise are in preventing strokes," says Ruiter, of the University of Alabama in Birmingham. "The public is less aware of the impact of insufficient amounts of sleep. Sleep is important — the body is stressed when it doesn't get the right amount."

Strokes occur when blood to the brain is restricted or cut off. Stroke is still the fourth-leading cause of death in the USA. Smoking, being overweight and inactivity are key risk factors.

The American Academy of Sleep Medicine seems to agree as noted in EurekAlert!

Top risk of stroke for normal-weight adults: Getting under 6 hours of sleep

Habitually sleeping less than six hours a night significantly increases the risk of stroke symptoms among middle-age to older adults who are of normal weight and at low risk for obstructive sleep apnea (OSA), according to a study of 5,666 people followed for up to three years.

After adjusting for body-mass index (BMI), they found a strong association with daily sleep periods of less than six hours and a greater incidence of stroke symptoms for middle-age to older adults, even beyond other risk factors. The study found no association between short sleep periods and stroke symptoms among overweight and obese participants.

"In employed middle-aged to older adults, relatively free of major risk factors for stroke such as obesity and sleep-disordered breathing, short sleep duration may exact its own negative influence on stroke development," said lead author Megan Ruiter, PhD. "We speculate that short sleep duration is a precursor to other traditional stroke risk factors, and once these traditional stroke risk factors are present, then perhaps they become stronger risk factors than sleep duration alone."

Be Inspired

6/18/12   Wow! Both Mother's Day and Father's Day have slipped by. Please be aware that if one of your biological parents has CKD, you are at higher risk for the disease. AND if you are the biological parent, so are your children. That made me so angry when it was ex-plained to me. Of course, I had no clue why I was angry – but it is said that anger is the flip side of sadness. I have children.

Some readers were surprised to discover that I'd seen my nutritionist not once, but twice annually. My nephrology center includes a yearly consultation with a nutritionist. Now that I'm older and on Medicare, I de-cided to see what they cover. Surprise! Three visits, the first year and two every year thereafter. This is from their website.

Medical Nutrition Therapy - How often is it covered?

Medicare covers medical nutrition therapy services prescribed by a doctor for people with diabetes or kidney disease. This benefit includes:
- An initial assessment of nutrition and lifestyle assessment
- Nutrition counseling
- Information regarding managing lifestyle factors that affect diet
- Follow-up visits to monitor progress managing diet

Medicare covers 3 hours of one-on-one counseling ser-vices the first year, and 2 hours each year after that. If your condition, treatment, or diagnosis changes, you may be able to get more hours of treatment with a doctor's referral. A doctor must prescribe these ser-vices and renew their referral yearly if you need treat-ment into another calendar year. These services can be given by a registered dietitian or Medicare approved nutrition professional.

Hopefully, this has inspired you to call your nephrologist for a visit with the practice's nutritionist. Let's move from using renal nutrition therapy to stave off End Stage Renal Disease to alternatives should you reach stage 5. What if you're among the 20% of CKDers who aren't able to stabilize at stage 3 and need to go on to dialysis? This article from the University of Washington caught my eye a couple of months ago. Frankly, I had trouble believing this was even possible. It just sounded too much like science fiction. After pondering and pondering, I'm now convinced it is more science than fiction. I'd be interested to hear your opinion.

Wearable artificial kidney to be tested for safety and effectiveness in collaboration with FDA
By Leila Gray and Linda Sellers

A wearable artificial kidney, designed as a new treatment for kidney failure, will be tested in Seattle. The trial will be done in collaboration with the Food and Drug Administration under a new Innovations Pathway announced Monday. The battery-powered wearable artificial kidney in its current form weighs about 10 pounds and is worn in a belt around the waist. Dr. Victor Gura, an associate clinical professor at the David Geffen School of Medicine, University of California, Los Angeles, invented the device. His goal is to free end-stage kidney disease patients from being tethered for several hours for three or more days a week to a dialysis machine. The hope is to improve the quality of life of these patients. Researchers will be testing a wearable device that takes over the blood-cleaning functions of the kidneys…. The Wearable Artificial Kidney is being developed by Blood Purification Technologies Inc. based in Beverly Hills, Calif.

"Quality of life issues will likely be embedded in the trial design," Himmelfarb said. "We'll probably be asking patients, 'Can you move with ease? How do you feel? How does the device or the treatment affect your daily life? Can you go to work with it on or go out with your family and friends?' We will be looking at key health outcomes as well as health economics."

"At present, if you want to attend your cousin's wedding in New York City, you need to check to be sure time slots are available at a center for you to get your dialysis done. You can't just walk in," he said. "If you live in a rural area, you probably drive a long distance every week for your dialysis sessions. A safe, effective, wearable artificial kidney would give end-stage kidney disease patients much more freedom in their lives."

So we've gone from renal nutritional therapy to external artificial kidneys in just one blog. I am so inspired to realize just how much is available to us.

It's All Connected

6/25/12 A friend suffered a really bad bout of gout recently: fever, extreme pain in his knees, loss of appetite, the whole gamut. That got me to thinking about what it would have meant to him if he had Chronic Kidney Disease. Researching that brought me to an English article from Arthritis Research UK which cited an American study. I'm going to reproduce only one paragraph of the article here because it brought home exactly what gout with Chronic Kidney Disease can do to your body.

The findings were presented at Kidney Week 2011 by researcher Dr Erdal Sarac. He concluded: "This study reveals a high prevalence of gout in patients with CKD. Male sex, advanced age, CAD, hypertension, and hyperlipidemia were significantly associated with gout among CKD patients."

In case you haven't got a copy of ***What Is It and How Did I Get It? Early Stage Chronic Kidney Disease*** handy, I've included a small glossary defining the terms in that last, information packed sentence.

CAD: coronary artery disease
gout: particularly painful form of inflammatory arthritis characterized by a build-up of urate crystals in the joints, causing pain and inflammation
hyperlipidemia: high cholesterol
hypertension: high blood pressure
urate: a salt of uric acid

One disease, CKD, can be implicated for three others if you also have gout. When I wrote about being careful what drugs your dentist gives you because you are already medically compromised by simply having CKD, I didn't know that gout is also somehow in the mix of being medically compromised.

I have hyperlipidemia and hypertension and CKD. True, I'm not an older male but should I become more vigilant about any hints of gout? I saw the pain my friend endured and don't want that for myself. I would have to be careful about my food and beverage intake.

Oh, wait, I'm already doing that by following the renal diet. In both, you are urged to cut back on alcohol and drink more water instead. Purines are a problem, too, but then again I am limited to five ounces of protein {A purine food source} per day. Hmmm, avoiding sugar-sweetened drinks may help. Say, with CKD, I have to watch my A1C {How the body handles glucose or sugar in a three month period} so that I don't end up with diabetes. That means I'm watching all my sugar intake already. I see fructose rich fruits can be a problem. But I'm already restricted to only three servings of fruit a day! Oh, here's the biggie: lose weight. Yep, been hearing that from my nephrologist for four years.

To sum up, by attending to my CKD on a daily basis, I'm also attempting to avoid or lessen the effects of gout. This is getting very interesting. I also take medication for both hypertension and hyperlipidemia. Are they also helping me to avoid gout? It seems to me that by treating one condition {Or two in my case}, I'm also treating my CKD and possibly preventing another. It is all inter-related.

This is part of an article from one of DaVita's sites. Notice how much of this advice overlaps that given to a gout patient.

Depending on what stage of Chronic Kidney Disease you're in, your renal dietitian will adjust the amounts of protein, sodium, phosphorus and potassium in your diet. In addition, carbohydrates and fats may be controlled based on conditions such as diabetes and cardiovascular disease. The CKD non-dialysis diet includes calculated amounts of high quality protein. Damaged kidneys have a difficult time getting rid of protein waste products, so cutting back on non-essential protein will put less stress on your kidneys.

Studies confirm that keeping your blood pressure in check can help slow the progression of kidney disease, especially if you have diabetes and/or proteinuria {Protein in the urine}. According to the National Kidney Foundation (NKF) guidelines, you should keep your blood pressure at or below 130/85 if you have kidney disease, and at or below 125/75 if you also have diabetes and/or proteinuria. Along with taking your prescribed blood pressure medications, lifestyle changes such as losing weight, exercising, meditating, eating less sodium, drinking less alcohol and quitting smoking can help lower blood pressure. Better blood pressure control helps preserve kidney function. If you have diabetes, tighter management of your blood glucose level can help slow the progression of kidney disease. It is important to keep your hemoglobin A1C at less than 6.5% or at the level established with your doctor, and closely monitor your blood glucose to avoid hypo-glycemia. Ask your doctor or diabetes educator about your diabetes treatment goals and options.

Regenerative Medicine or Last Year's Science Fiction Becomes the Future's Science

7/2/12   July 4th, Independence Day, is Wednesday. There's another kind of independence down the pike for us – independence from the dialysis that is the only alternative now for ESRD sufferers. Okay, now get ready to be amazed and learn a new word.

Podocytes are found only in the kidney and are an integral structural component of its blood-filtering system. They stand shoulder-to-shoulder in a part of the organ called the glomerulus {As CKD patients, that word should be more than familiar} and wrap their long 'feet' {Pod is Greek for foot, just as ped is Latin for foot.} A-round the semi-permeable capillaries through which blood flows. Narrow slits between the feet allow small molecules, such as water and salts, to pass while block-ing large proteins {Sound familiar?}....

"The implication is that podocytes may utilize recog-nized pathways of regeneration to renew themselves throughout life," said Artandi (associate professor of medicine Steven Artandi, MD, PhD. and senior author of the study). People suffering from Chronic Kidney Dis-ease {That's us.} may simply have worn out or outpaced their podocytes' capacity for renewal, he believes.

Now that the researchers know podocytes have the ability {to} regenerate in response to common cellular signals, their next step is to learn whether this regen-eration occurs in healthy animals and people. "If we can harness this regeneration," Artandi said, "we may one day be able to treat people with Chronic Kidney Disease."

According to the article, there is a possibility in the future of coaxing our own bodies to produce more of these podocytes to replace those that have died. This is another new way of treating Chronic Kidney Disease. Add this to cloning, artificial kidneys, external mechanical kidneys and the future holds just so many more options than three different types of dialysis. I, for one, am so encouraged I can feel my heart leaping in my chest {Well, maybe not, but I am super encouraged.}.

In the same vein {Get it? Medical term? Vein?}, are you aware that kidneys can be 3D printed? I had to read that sentence twice myself. Then I started – why even bother making a 3D print of a kidney. Read on as Wake Forest University's Anthony Atala explains.

"….For example, the talk highlights our still-experimental work to engineer a human kidney. Being able to replace solid organs such as the heart, liver, kidney {Note that – kidney.} and pancreas is considered the "holy grail" of tissue engineering. That's why we're pursuing multiple strategies in this area: cell therapies, tissue "inserts" to augment an organ's function, and "printing" replacement organs.

At TED {TED stands for Technology, Entertainment Design.}, we demonstrated 3-D printing technology, already used in a variety of industries — from auto parts to concrete structures. Our goal, or course, is to apply the technology to organs. The project is based on earlier research in which we engineered miniature kidneys {Hurray!} using biomaterials and cells. In animals, these structures were shown to be functional, in that they were able to filter blood and produce dilute urine.

This printer, while still experimental, is being explored for organs such as the kidney {Ahem.} and structured tissue such as the ear. The ultimate goal is to use patient data, such as from a CT scan, to create a computer model of the organ we want to print. This model would be used to guide the printer as it layer-by-layer prints a replacement organ made up of cells and the biomaterials to hold the cells together.

The FDA is on board, too, with their Innovation Pathway program which was launched in 2010 to reduce the time and cost of bringing safe and effective breakthrough technologies to patients. These three aimed at kidney patients were approved earlier this year:

- An implantable Renal Assist Device being developed by the University of California, San Francisco.
- A Wearable Artificial Kidney in development by Blood Purification Technologies Inc. of Beverly Hills, Calif. {Discussed in a blog last month.}
- A Hemoaccess Valve System that has been designed by Greenville, S.C.-based CreatiVasc Medical.

Better and Better

7/9/12 The estimated glomerular filtration rate as the norm for evaluating the presence – and stage of – Chronic Kidney Disease may change. Now you take a blood test and you catch your urine for 24 hours, right? Then it's tested.

Here's where the change may happen. Currently, only the creatinine is evaluated -not the creatinine and cystatin-c. The what, you say? Good question and one I had to research myself.

According to medterms.com:

It is a serum protein that is filtered out of the blood by the kidneys and that serves as a measure of kidney function.

A National Institute of Health study found that testing both creatinine and cystatin-c is more accurate which could prevent over diagnosing CKD and, more importantly to me, missing the CKD.

By the way, I found some interesting articles about this dated as far back as five years ago. I'm wondering why our nephrologists have not yet changed the tests they request to test for CKD.

Good, Bad or Unnecessary?

7/16/12   I had this crazy desire to clean, although the house in pristine condition. I tried to ignore it, but that didn't work. So, I cleaned, right down to cleaning out the articles I keep for the blog. Of course, being me, I had to read each one before I trashed it. Lo and behold, I started seeing a pattern with some of them. On Halloween of last year, this article appeared. By the end of the blog, you'll be able to figure out if it was a trick or a treat.

FDA staff say Merck's Vytorin helps kidney patients

U.S. Food and Drug Administration reviewers said Merck's cholesterol-lowering drug Vytorin was effective in reducing the rate of heart attacks or other cardio-vascular problems in patients with kidney disease. The FDA reviewers also said Merck's blockbuster drug, which pairs a new type of cholesterol fighter Zetia with Merck's older statin drug Zocor, is unlikely to cause or promote cancer.

But, as I read further in the article, I found that Vytorin contained the generic drug simvastatin which had already been approved to lower cholesterol. Something nagged at me, so I went to Drugs.com to check out Vytorin. This is what I found there.

What is Vytorin?

Vytorin contains a combination of ezetimibe and simvastatin. Vytorin is used to treat high cholesterol in adults and children who are at least 10 years old. Ezetimibe reduces the amount of cholesterol absorbed by the body. Simvastatin is in a group of drugs called HMG CoA reductase inhibitors, or "statins." Simvastatin reduces levels of "bad" cholesterol (low-density lipoprotein, or LDL) and triglycerides in the blood, while increasing levels of "good" cholesterol (high-density lipoprotein, or HDL). {Another of Vytorin's original claims had been that it attacks both genetic and life habit causes of hyperlipidemia. Remember those TV ads about whether what you ate or Uncle Frank's genes caused your high cholesterol? That's where this claim was made.}

As I kept reading, I found two disturbing warnings.

1. In rare cases, simvastatin can cause a condition that results in the breakdown of skeletal muscle tissue, lead-ing to kidney failure. This condition may be more like-ly to occur in older adults and in people who have kidney disease or poorly controlled hypothyroidism (underactive thyroid).

2. Avoid eating foods that are high in fat or cholesterol. Vytorin will not be as effective in lowering your cholesterol if you do not follow a cholesterol-lowering diet plan.

So a pill that combats high cholesterol on both fronts – genetics and life habits – still requires a life habit change {Diet} but could kill CKD patients when given to them to avoid heart problems. I was not happy. But it gets even weirder. Remember that simvastatin supposedly lowers bad cholesterol and raises good cholesterol and that simvastatin is the generic drug in Vytorin.

**'Good' cholesterol's heart benefits challenged
Drugs to raise HDL can't be assumed to reduce heart attack risk**

Having naturally high levels of "good" cholesterol doesn't lower the risk of heart attacks as believed. LDL cholesterol is referred to as "bad" cholesterol because when there's too much, it promotes the build-up of plaque in artery walls.

HDL cholesterol is known as "good" cholesterol because higher concentrations have been associated with lower risk of heart attacks in observational studies. The hoped for benefits of increasing high-density lipoprotein or HDL cholesterol for lowering heart attack risk haven't panned out in randomized trials of experimental drugs. According to conventional wisdom, those who inherit genetic variants for higher HDL levels should have lower cardiovascular risk. When researchers tested 116,000 people, they found 2.6 per cent of them were genetically predisposed to have higher concentrations of HDL."

So you may be taking a drug prescribed to treat your hyperlipidemia but it doesn't matter if your good cholesterol is raised, even though that's one of Merck's {The manufacturer} claims. In addition, it is possible that this drug prescribed to prevent heart problems in CKD patients may kill them. Why do I get the sinking feeling that this is business as usual for the drug industry?

Whatever Happened to Common Sense?

7/23/12   There are two different severe medical emergencies in the family right now. Both of these beloved people are in hospitals, two different hospitals in two different states. I looked at the menu of the one in an Arizona hospital and realized that, while this unrestricted diet was tasty and enticing, it was sodium laden. That reminded me of a Canadian study about the sodium content of hospital food there that I'd read recently on CBC News. It's an eye opener and made me wonder about just plain common sense.

Hospital meals need to hold the salt
Prepared, processed foods often too high in sodium

Hospital patients get too much salt even when they're on a sodium restricted diet, says a Canadian study. On average, Canadians consume 3,400 milligrams of sodium a day, which is 1,100 milligrams over the recommended levels. At least three-quarters of that sodium comes from processed foods.

Restricting sodium is particularly important for certain hospital patients, such as those with heart failure. Re-gistered dietitian and postdoctoral researcher JoAnne Arcand of the University of Toronto and her colleagues and Mount Sinai Hospital analyzed 84 standard menus for regular, diabetic and sodium-restricted diets at three hospitals in Ontario between 2010 and 2011.

"We demonstrated that hospital patient menus contain excessive levels of sodium," the study's authors concluded in a letter published in Monday's online issue of the *Archives of Internal Medicine*.

This, in turn, reminded me of another article I'd read that seemed somewhat unnecessary since I'd thought it was just common sense. Maybe it isn't. Basically the article discussed the salt content of fast foods and how that pertains to CKD patients.

Salt Intake and Hypertension – the plot thickens....

There is good evidence to support a connection between salt intake and population-based blood pressure levels. Excess dietary salt is associated with increased blood pressure in individuals. It has also been argued that like the effects of restraining tobacco consumption there would also be a salutary effect on population outcomes if salt intake was constrained.

A recent article in the June 12 issue of CMAJ by Elizabeth Dunford and colleagues is a must-read because of its practical importance. Basically, Dunford and co-workers performed a survey assessing the salt content of food items sold by 6 trans-national food companies operating in the US, Australia, Canada, France, New Zealand, and the UK. They calculated mean salt content and compared these within and between countries and companies. The companies involved were: Burger King (known as Hungry Jack's in Australia), Domino's Pizza, Kentucky Fried Chicken, McDonald's, Pizza Hut and Subway....

The authors conclude: "Decreasing salt in fast foods

would appear to be technically feasible and is likely to produce important gains in population health — the mean salt levels of fast foods are high, and these foods are eaten often. Governments setting and enforcing salt targets for industry would provide a level playing field, and no company could gain a commercial advantage by using high levels of salt."

The other practical point, of course, is that when we see patients with CKD who invariably have hypertension that is difficult to control, we should educate them about salt content in fast food items and how much variability there currently is.

I simply could not accept that we were as senseless as these two articles seemed to indicate, so I mined all the articles I'd saved about sodium and thankfully came up to this one from *Primary Issues*. It's clear and offers you some control about the sodium in your life.

According to CDC {That's the Centers for Disease Control and Prevention.} Director Thomas Frieden, MD, "Too much sodium raises blood pressure, which is a major risk factor for heart disease and stroke. These diseases kill more than 800,000 Americans each year and contribute an estimated $273 billion in healthcare costs."

But nutritionists believe that salt poured at the table is rarely the culprit in sending Americans past the threshold, because eaters can more easily control the salt shaker at home; it's the hidden salt found in many processed foods, or in meals eaten outside the home, that help push Americans over the limits. CDC estimates that reducing the sodium content of the 10 leading sodium sources by 25% would lower total dietary sodium by more than 10% and could play a role in preventing up to an estimated 28,000 deaths per year.

The article contained a chart and suggestions that made it simple to understand table salt is not the culprit. Here we are congratulating ourselves for banishing the salt shaker from our tables only to discover it's the salt INSIDE the foods we eat that does much damage, too.

Why the Book?

7/30/12   Some of you are already aware of the severe, non-renal, medical emergencies which have occurred in my family during the last two weeks. For those of you who aren't, one of the emergencies deals with diabetes-hypertension-possible cancer-mental health. The other is purely mental health. Before I got the chance to try to calm my loved ones a little by reminding each of them that everything happens for a reason, whether or not we know the reason, they reminded me. And, as usual, that got me to thinking....

I have been asked repeatedly why I wrote **What Is It and How Did I Get It? Early Stage Chronic Kidney Disease.** You'd expect that question on the radio health shows I guested on and it was there. You'd also expect that question at the renal symposium, book signings and book talks I was involved with and, yes, it was there too. But when I most often hear the question is when I'm just chatting with friends, theirs friends, someone's family – you know, ordinary, everyday people like you or me.

I've carefully explained each time I'm asked. Then I happened upon an article at DaVita that said the same thing with more authority than I could ever muster. I know we usually think of DaVita in association with End Stage Renal Disease, but they have a wonderfully comforting educational unit to their website as well. I kept running into this article whenever I was researching. Since I do believe everything happens for a reason, whether or not we know the reason, I figured that I was meant to share it with you via the blog. These are the parts of the article that hit home for me as far as why I wrote the book.

It can be overwhelming to discover you have Chronic Kidney Disease. Sometimes the amount of new information seems mind-boggling, but it's important for you to remain calm. You may feel like you're losing control, but in fact, you are the key to maintaining your health. You, above any doctor, nurse or dietitian, are the head of your kidney disease health care team. {The book was written from my feeling overwhelmed and not wanting any other CKD patient to feel that way.}

The one person who has been an intimate part of your health care since day one is you. You know how you feel when you get the flu, you know how your body responds to medicine, you know if you're allergic to something, and you've known yourself your whole life. Now that you are dealing with kidney disease, your job has become even more important.

If you feel confident being your own kidney disease health care advocate, be sure to cover all your questions and concerns by making a checklist. The best way to tackle issues is to keep a pad of paper handy and when you think of things you want to discuss with your doctor, jot them down. On your next doctor's visit take out your pad and cross each item off after you address it. Your medical team will be impressed, and you will also get more out of your visit. {It is important to get those answers. ***What Is It and How Did I Get It? Early Stage Chronic Kidney Disease*** will help you formulate the questions. That was my problem. I wanted answers, but I didn't know the questions to ask.}

If you have a pressing concern that won't wait until your next doctor's appointment, feel free to call your doctor, nurse practitioner or renal dietitian. You can also start researching your question on davita.com. DaVita offers a comprehensive and easy to use website that specializes in renal {Kidney} education.

It's always a good idea to follow your kidney doctor's advice. {But ask WHY they've given you this advice and make sure you understand it rather than blindly doing as you're told. It's quite an unfair burden on your doctor, too, when you do as you're told without taking any responsibility.} They have gone to medical school, seen many patients and chosen a career to help people with kidney disease.

While doctors are loaded with medical information, they are people first. Doctors may assume you understand everything when you don't, they may not be aware of personal situations, and sometimes they don't have all the answers. {Bingo! There's my reason in a nutshell.} That's why you need to be the head of your kidney disease health care team. The kidney doctors, nurses and renal dietitians are on your health care team, and you are a key player in that team. If something's not right, you must consult your health care team to find a solution. If you're unclear on anything regarding your treatment or kidney disease care, ask again. Your health is the priority of your team and when you succeed, so do they.

The State of the Mind Address

8/6/12   One of my children is being successfully treated for depression and anxiety, but has developed a pre-diabetic condition and elevated cholesterol. So, what did I do? What else? I researched mental life's effect on physical health. I found information I'd always taken for granted proven scientifically and some – like the different types of smiles – I hadn't thought about. I zeroed in on the following in one of the articles I found.

Poor mental health linked to reduced life expectancy

There is a possibility that mental health problems may be associated with biological changes in the body that increase the risk of diseases such as heart disease. In this study, approximately a quarter of people suffered from minor symptoms of anxiety and depression, however, these patients do not usually come to the attention of mental health services. The authors say that their findings could have implications for the way minor mental health problems are treated. It made sense to me.

Another one of my children had troublesomely high cholesterol when she was agonizing over a major life decision three years ago. She took her medication, ate the right foods and made certain she exercised and it kept right on rising. Fast forward to a few months after she made and acted upon her decision.

She faced her fear and returned to her doctor for a complete physical even though she had stopped taking the medication and ignored her diet. As a dancer (She *is* my daughter}, exercise wasn't a problem. I'm so glad she did go back to the doctor. There is no sign of ele- vated cholesterol. Why? I'm laying it on the fact that she's happier now.

I tend to smile quite a bit and look for reasons to smile even when life seems hard. I wondered if that were helping me with my own health and, if so, would it help others. Then I located this Aug. 1, MNT article.

Smiling Reduces Stress And Helps The Heart

A new study suggests that holding a smile on one's face during periods of stress may help the heart. The study, due to be published in a forthcoming issue of *Psych-ological Science*, lends support to the old adage 'grin and bear it,' suggesting it may also make us feel better.

Oh, got an email from a reader whose tests showed she had NO CKD, although she'd been diagnosed at stage 3. Being a smart one, she retook the tests. The first set of tests had false results. No one knows quite how that happened, but if you should find you suddenly have test results, good or bad, that are totally unexpected, please have them redone. We all want NOT to have CKD, but need to pay attention to it if we do.

To Sleep: Perchance to Dream

8/13/12   First: credit where credit is due. Thanks to the Bard, William Shakespeare, for providing the title for today's blog. Anyone recognize it from Hamlet's soliloquy?

Although I'd planned to write about my odd experience with the threat of heart disease {It turned out to be some ridiculous fluke in the machinery.} in next week's blog, people have already started asking what heart disease has to do with Chronic Kidney Disease.

The American Association of Kidney Patients has an easily understood, comprehensive article about just that. This statement sums it up in a nutshell:

"Individuals with kidney disease are at a high risk of developing hardening of the arteries resulting in heart attacks, heart failure and strokes."

In addition, although I am not astute enough to completely understand the studies I read about women and EKG testing, there does seem to be conclusive evidence that the female heart *is* more sensitive to the EKG and could provide a false positive for heart disease. Phew! I feel like I dodged a bullet on that one.

So, what is today's blog topic? Sleep! If you remember, I'd had a sleep study just before the EKG panic but never got to write about sleep apnea and CKD. You should know that I'd spent over four years trying to convince my nephrologist that I was tired because the CKD prevented me from producing enough red blood cells and he spent the same amount of time trying to convince me that wasn't why I was always so tired.

In retrospect, it's surprising that neither one of us ever considered sleep apnea. It wasn't until one of my many daughters was diagnosed with OSA that I started wondering if I could have it. Of course, then I spent some time wondering if I were going to consider myself a victim of whatever health problem anyone I knew had. Once I got beyond that, help was on the way. I found a study in which sleep apnea and hypertension are clearly linked:

"We think there may be a causative factor here; that sleep apnea may be causing direct glomerular injury," Dr John J Sim (Kaiser Permanente, Los Angeles, CA) told renal*wire* . "We already know that sleep apnea causes hypertension and that hypertension causes kidney disease."

If some degree of causality can be shown, it's possible that treating sleep apnea may slow the progression of kidney disease, the authors speculate.

This is an older study from 2005, but it seems to lead the way to further proof that sleep apnea does affect CKD. It's also the only one I could understand {Sometimes I do wish I were a doctor.} which even mentions glomerular injury. I think we need a definition of sleep apnea – also called obstructive sleep apnea or OSA – before we go any further, preferably a non-medicalese one. The simplest definition I could locate is from Yahoo! Health.

"sleep apnea is a condition in which a person has episodes of blocked breathing during sleep."

I should add the episodes usually last 10 seconds or longer. During those episodes, you wake yourself up by gasping or snorting in an effort to start breathing again. Now that I understand exactly what is happening, it's sort of scary. I hadn't realized this could be serious. But, being me, I'm not going to let it. Hence, the sleep study.

You don't just walk into a sleep center to request one of these. My family doctor referred me to several pulmonologists, lung and respiratory tract specialists. After I chose one, she suggested a sleep study. Off I went to make my appointment.

While they did a terrific job of monitoring my sleep patterns during different sleep states, I was unimpressed. I don't know what I expected, but they hooked me up, sent me to sleep, then woke me up to put on a CPAP and sent me back to sleep.

According to WiseGeek.com:

A CPAP machine has a small box connected to tubes through which air flows. The tubes are connected to a mask worn on the face. Straps around the mask fit it to the face over the mouth and nose. For those with sleep apnea, the CPAP is used at night during normal sleep.

A CPAP was recommended for me. I am not thrilled and made it clear I'd like to try an oral {Sometimes called dental.} device to see how effective that is before I agreed to the CPAP. I have reservations about being hooked up to a machine. Those are my personal reservations. Many, many people are perfectly comfortable with the CPAP.

Stressed? You Must Be Kidding

8/21/12   While talking to my cardiologist, he men-
tioned the stellar reviews for **What Is It and How
Did I Get It? Early Stage Chronic Kidney Disease** on
Amazon. Talk about being surprised!

Back to the much more important cardiology information. There is no, zero, zilch history of heart disease in
my family BUT {as we all know}, I do have Chronic
Kidney Disease. That moves me up a notch for developing heart problems.

According to the U.S. National Library of Medicine, CKD
may be the cause of the following heart and blood
vessel complications:

- Congestive heart failure
- Coronary artery disease
- High blood pressure
- Pericarditis
- Stroke

I was worried, but keeping my fear under control. Here's
what happened. I needed pre-op clearance for the cataract surgery. My trustworthy primary care doctor {PCP}
was unavailable, so her lovely and efficient Physician's
Assistant made an appointment for me with the nurse
practitioner {NP} in the practice. This woman asked her
own physician assistant to perform an EKG on me –
twice since she didn't like the results of the first one.

I didn't know the NP, but was more than a bit discon-

certed that she arrived late, had not looked at the notes, did not believe me when I pointed out on the ophthalmologist's request that I needed an EKG, and asked my PCP's PA {Physician's Assistant} to verify, and – here's the worst one – was visibly shaken at the EKG
results.

Okay, maybe I was annoyed when I walked in {None of this was taken care of in a timely fashion despite my phone calls so it ended up being a terrific rush}, but if anyone should be upset at the results, shouldn't it be the patient?

The practice provided cardiology recommendations since it was clear seeing one was my next step. I called the closest one hoping they could get me in before my scheduled surgery. I was in the next day. Every single one of my numerous questions was answered and a stress test scheduled for the next day after reading the results of the EKG I'd been given in this office.

The cardiologist wandered into the examining room while I was there and explained that EKGs can be inter-preted from different aspects. While the NP used elec-trodes on many different parts of my body, the card-iologist concentrated on those areas nearer the heart. These EKG results were far less worrisome, but there still was an abnormality in one part of my heart function they wanted to explore. Hence, the stress test.

I was made very comfortable during that test and even supplied a blanket since nuclear medicine rooms need to be kept very cold. I was injected with a slightly radioactive dye, but was assured this went nowhere near the kidneys and was so safe that I didn't even have to check with the nephrologist about its use.

The test results came back normal. According to the cardiologist, an EKG may be too sensitive to female hearts. I'm having trouble verifying that via research, but I have to admit I had no symptoms and no results. I wonder why the NP didn't explain that so I wouldn't worry about the possible diagnoses {Infarction, which means heart attack, was one of them.} on the EKG print out she gave me.

Moral: Go to doctors you know or have an immediate affinity with. I didn't know any of these doctors, but was immediately frustrated with the NP, while I immediately felt comfortable with the cardiologist.

Is this sound medical advice? Hardly, but it makes me feel better should I have to see that doctor again. Of course, if you have no affinity with someone who is the best doctor for you, ignore my advice. I've done that myself. The nice thing about advice is that you don't have to take it.

So Is It A Good Thing or Not?

8/27/12   I cannot begin to tell you how eager I am for the second cataract surgery. The repaired eye sees so well that the other one seems worse than it really is. In my big ten minutes of reading at a time while the repaired eye continues to heal, I've seen the same word over and over again. It isn't a word I usually expect to see: statin. According to Macmillandictionary.com, it means

a drug that is used to reduce the amount of cholesterol in the blood. This class of drugs can have a different name in other countries. It performs its miracle by inhibiting a key enzyme while encouraging the receptor binding of LDL-cholesterol {Low-density lipoprotein which causes health problems and cardiovascular dis-
ease}, resulting in decreased levels of serum cholesterol {That's cholesterol in the blood stream.} and LDL-cholesterol and increased levels of HDL-cholesterol.

I don't know about you, but I went running back to *What Is It and How Did I Get It? Early Stage Chronic Kidney Disease* to remind myself what that all means. From the glossary, I understood that dyslipidemia means abnormal levels of cholesterol, triglycerides or both. Well then, what does HDL-cholesterol do?

What else? This so called good cholesterol fights LDL-cholesterol. This is important because what we call the bad cholesterol {LDL-cholesterol} can build up in your arteries and may even block them eventually. Look at page 97 in the book for a clear diagram of just how this affects your blood pressure.

Let's get to the articles now. One from The American Medical Association this past June suggests that statins may cause fatigue and that women may experience this more than men. Notice the mention of vitamin D production in the article.

Study links statin use to fatigue
One possible reason is that reducing cholesterol levels can lead to the production of less vitamin D. All right, I'm a woman. I take statins. I'm fatigued, but I take vitamin D supplements. Back to the sleep apnea exploration for me.

Then in July, only one month later, this article appeared in *The New York Times*.

Women May Benefit Less From Statins
Many studies have found that statins reduce the risk for recurring cardiac problems, but not the risk for death. Now an analysis suggests that the drugs may reduce mortality significantly only in men.

Back in February of this year, *The New York Times* was warning us about the possible side effects of statins, albeit rare ones.

Safety Alerts Cite Cholesterol Drugs' Side Effects
Federal health officials on Tuesday added new safety alerts to the prescribing information for statins, the cholesterol-reducing medications that are among the most widely prescribed drugs in the world, citing rare risks of memory loss, diabetes and muscle pain.

Hmmm, my primary care doctor has been monitoring me for muscle pain since we met. She has already changed my statins three times in the last five years. As for the memory loss, who can tell? I'm at that age, you know.

Diabetes can be a problem. You take statins to reduce your LDL cholesterol so that you don't end up with high blood pressure, but it may cause diabetes. Which is the lesser of the two evils? Read on for help from USA Today this month to make that decision.

Benefits of cholesterol-cutting drugs outweigh diabetes risk

The benefits of taking cholesterol-lowering med-ications outweigh the increased risk some patients have of developing diabetes from using the drugs, a report out Thursday says.

Patients who were at higher risk for diabetes were 39% less likely to develop a cardiovascular illness on statins and 17% less likely to die. Patients who were not already at risk for diabetes and were taking statins had a 52% reduction in cardiovascular illness, and no increase in diabetes risk.

"When we focus only on the risk (of diabetes) we may be doing a disservice to our patients," says lead author Paul Ridker of Brigham and Women's Hospital in Boston. "As it turns out for this data, the hazard of being on a statin is limited almost entirely to those well on their way to getting diabetes."

Also this month, there was good news about statins.

Statins reduce pancreatitis risk

Statins reduce the risk for pancreatitis in patients with normal or mildly elevated triglyceride levels, say the authors of a large meta-analysis.

My all-time favorite appeared in *The New York Times* as blog in March of this year.

Do Statins Make It Tough to Exercise?

For years, physicians and scientists have been aware that statins, the most widely prescribed drugs in the world, can cause muscle aches and fatigue in some patients. What many people don't know is that these side effects are especially pronounced in people who exercise.

I got this smug sense of satisfaction at a hit against gallbladderkeep my organs healthy. Damned if you do; damned if you don't.

Being in the midst of cataract surgeries, I could not help myself. I had to include this month's article from MNT even though it doesn't mention CKD.

Cataracts Risk Associated With Statins

A new study, appearing in the August issue of

Optometry and Vision Science, has found that patients might have an increased risk of developing age-related cataracts if they use cholesterol-lowering statin drugs.

Oh, Say Can You See?

9/3/12   My own cataract surgery got me to thinking if this was in any way related to my Chronic Kidney Disease. In a Google search, this is the first site that came up – my old friend DaVita.

Eyes and Chronic Kidney Disease

The leading causes of Chronic Kidney Disease (CKD) are diabetes and high blood pressure. These conditions are also the leading causes of eye disease and loss of vision. If your renal disease is a result of either condition your vision may be at risk. Diabetes and high blood pressure often go undiagnosed because people don't notice any symptoms. As time goes on without medical treatment, these conditions can worsen and other complications—such as kidney disease and eye problems—arise. If you have Chronic Kidney Disease not due to high blood pressure you may still want to monitor your blood pressure regularly, as kidney disease can cause high blood pressure and put your vision at risk.

Cataracts

Cataracts occur when the lens of your eye becomes cloudy. The lens of the eye is normally clear. Its purpose is to focus the light coming in from the pupil to the retina at the back of the eye. A cataract scatters the incoming light and can make everything look blurry. Cataracts develop as we age. But patients with diabetes are at a higher risk for cataracts. Diabetics can develop what is known as "sugar cataracts," a cataract that appears suddenly and grows to such a point that the entire lens is clouded. High levels of glucose react with proteins found in the eye and form a byproduct that settles on the lens.

Hmmm, I don't have diabetes but I do have high blood pressure {Oh, okay, and I'm old – scratch that and make it older}. Let me describe the surgery to you.

There was the usual fasting as of midnight the previous night and the wait broken up by filling out forms and watching videos about post op care. Almost forgot: I was told to take only my hypertension medication and no others.

Then I was escorted into the pre op area where the usual vitals were taken and I was put out for a few minutes while the substance to paralyze the eye was injected directly into the eye. In retrospect, I'm glad I didn't have to suffer that wide awake.

But the surgery itself was an incredible surprise. I knew I was going to be awake during the procedure but I was unprepared for the beautiful colors I would see through the eye. I had to be reminded to be quiet so that the talking wouldn't make my head move.

I wanted to know why I was seeing the enchanting turquoise auras around the ceiling lights. Then I became more interested in what I can only describe as turquoise circuit boards that I saw in that eye. I'm pretty sure that was the original lens being blasted to pieces. I distinctly remember losing interest during the insertion of the new lens.

This scientific explanation from All About Vision makes the procedure more clear.

"Most modern cataract procedures involve the use of a high-frequency ultrasound probe that breaks up the cloudy lens into small pieces, which are then gently removed from the eye with suction. This procedure, called phacoemulsification or 'phaco,' can be perform-ed with smaller incisions than previous surgical techniques for cataract removal, promoting faster healing and reducing the risk of cataract surgery complications, such as a retinal detachment.

After the cataract and all remnants of the cloudy lens have been removed from your eye, the cataract surgeon inserts a clear intraocular lens {You'll see that referred to as an IOL in the rest of the explanation.}, positioning it securely behind the iris and pupil, in the same location your natural lens occupied. (In special cases, an IOL might be placed in front of the iris and pupil, but this is less common.) The surgeon then completes the cataract removal and IOL implantation procedure by closing the incision in your eye (a stitch may or may not be needed), and a protective shield is placed over the eye to keep it safe in the early stages of your cataract surgery recovery."

The only complaint I had about the entire procedure was that the surgery table I was laying on had no shoulders making it uncomfortable after a while. This same table was rolled into the surgery room, so it made sense that the shoulder areas were cut out. That's so that the surgeon could pull his stool as close to my

eye as possible.

Here's the part you have to watch out for {I know, poor choice of words for describing cataract surgery}. Although I had carefully explained that I have Chronic Kidney Disease, I was still given a sulphur based medication to prevent pressure from accumulating in the recovering eye. If you've read ***What Is It and How Did I Get It? Early Stage Chronic Kidney Disease***, you know that this is not good for the kidneys and my nephrologist was very upset that they were given to me when I had a bladder infection a couple of years ago.

I talked this over with my ophthalmologist who seemed surprised that it was given to me and assured me I needn't take it after the second surgery. I hope I hadn't made a mistake by taking it after the first surgery, but when the nurse said BOTH my doctors prescribed it, I thought she meant the ophthalmologist and my nephrologist. As I sat there for the required hour for recovery before being released, I realized she'd meant the ophthalmologist and the anesthesiologist. Uh-oh, I'll have to keep a close eye {Sorry! I couldn't resist} on my numbers on my next labs.

Drink Up

9/10/12 Something kept nagging at me until I forced myself to remember what it was {Who knew humans had the capacity to do that?}. Something about what we drink. Since we, as Chronic Kidney Disease patients, barely – or in my case, never – imbibe that means juice, water or soft drinks. I'd rather get the fiber in my big three servings of fruit a day so that narrows the choice to water or soft drinks. That's what it was!

This is an older article from *Natural News*, but one that resonates even with those who insist upon drinking soda.

Aspartame alert: Diet soda destroys kidney function

Scientists from Brigham and Women's Hospital in Boston have revealed results from a study outlining some of the effects of artificial sweeteners on the body. Conducted on a group of 3,000 women, the results indicated that those who drank two or more artificially-sweetened beverages a day doubled their risk of more-rapid-than-normal kidney function decline.

The article includes the fact that more sodium is used in diet sodas, and how stevia {Natural sweetener} could be used instead.

The American Cancer Society seems to have only one concern about aspartame as of February of this year.

Wikipedia has this to say about aspartame.

Aspartame ... is an artificial, non-saccharide sweetener used as a sugar substitute in some foods and beverages. In the European Union, it is codified as E951. Aspartame is a methyl ester of the aspartic acid/phenylalanine dipeptide. It was first sold under the brand name NutraSweet; since 2009 it also has been sold under the brand name AminoSweet. It was first synthesized in 1965 and the patent expired in 1992.

The following is my favorite article by far. I am a coffee lover to the point that I sometimes buy and blend my own beans. Yes, of course I have Chronic Kidney Disease and, yes, of course caffeine is frowned upon, but there are those 16 oz. {Two whole cups!!!!} permitted for those who simply must have their coffee – me! Remember, I mention in **What Is It and How Did I Get It? EarlyStage Chronic Kidney Disease** that this helps keep me from feeling deprived since I follow the renal diet.

Kicking your morning off with a cup of Joe may provide more than a caffeine boost. A recent study from the National Institutes of Health (NIH) found that older coffee drinkers — even those who swill decaf — have a lower risk of death than those who don't drink coffee.

"Coffee is one of the most widely consumed beverages, both in the United States and worldwide," the authors of the study write. "Since coffee contains caffeine, a stimulant, coffee drinking is not generally considered to be part of a healthy lifestyle.

Howeverever, coffee is a rich source of antioxidants and other bioactive compounds. ”

Another article from CBC News in June of this year talks about water. While you read this, keep in mind that CKD folks need 64 ounces of FLUID, not necessarily water, a day.

8 glasses of water a day 'an urban myth'

Water and a well-balanced diet 'do far more than water alone,' Australian researcher says

The common advice to drink eight glasses of water a day doesn't hold water, say nutrition and kidney specialists who want to dispel the myth. The article includes fluid from other sources, including my beloved coffee.

The Coffee Blog

9/17/12 Last week's blog discussed different kinds of drinks. I mentioned that coffee is my favorite. Since I'm still recovering from the second cataract surgery and we all know how good it feels to be self-indulgent when you're recovering, this week's blog is all about coffee. I won't be repeating what I included in last week's blog, but there is quite a bit of medical information about coffee available. Let me just pour myself a cup and I'll tell you….

Here's what *the New York Times* had to say.

Really? Drinking Coffee Lowers Colon Cancer Risk
Over the years, most studies of the subject have been either small or plagued by methodological flaws. But recently a team of researchers at the National Cancer Institute followed half a million Americans over 15 years. The researchers looked in detail at their diets, habits and health, and found that people who drank four or more cups of coffee a day — regular or decaf — had a 15 percent lower risk of colon cancer compared with coffee abstainers.

While the researchers could not prove cause and effect, they did find that the link was dose-responsive: Greater coffee consumption was correlated with a lower colon cancer risk. The effect held even after they adjusted their findings for factors like exercise, family history of cancer, body weight, and alcohol and cigarette use.

And to answer your question about what colon cancer has to do with Chronic Kidney Disease, you have to remember you are medically compromised already. Cancer is a disease caused by inflammation, just as Chronic Kidney Disease is. By the way, it's said that alkaline foods are a better way of eating should cancer rear its ugly head in your life.

Coffee Drinking Linked to Lower Death Risk
Older adults who drank coffee—caffeinated or decaffeinated—had a lower risk of death overall than others who did not, according a study by researchers from the National Cancer Institute and AARP. Coffee drinkers were less likely to die from heart disease, respiratory disease, stroke, injuries and accidents, diabetes, and infections.

Thank you to the Robert Wood Johnson Foundation for that information.

I am an older {Thank you for that 'er'} adult. I absolutely love coffee. I also have Chronic Kidney Disease which may lead me down the primrose path to diabetes. Perhaps I can prevent that? Too bad I'm restricted to two cups a day.

This one from EurekAlert.org can get a bit technical so I've copied the most easily understood part of it:

Coffee consumption inversely associated with risk of most common form of skin cancer

Increasing the number of cups of caffeinated coffee

you drink could lower your risk of developing the most common form of skin cancer, basal cell carcinoma, according to a study published in *Cancer Research*, a journal of the American Association for Cancer Research.

"Our data indicate that the more caffeinated coffee you consume, the lower your risk of developing basal cell carcinoma," said Jiali Han, Ph.D., associate professor at Brigham and Women's Hospital, Harvard Medical School in Boston and Harvard School of Public Health. So coffee - formerly universally maligned by the medical community – now can help prevent colon and skin cancer and prolong your life.

I'm liking this very much, but we're not done, folks. I'm grinding {Love being punny} the sources out right now. I am in heaven! Look what I found at Everyday Health. You'll probably understand my over the top joy if you remember I've had both a root canal and a crown replacement so the dentist could reach the cavity underneath the crown this summer.

9 Healthy Reasons to Indulge Your Coffee Cravings

Coffee gets a bad rap, but study after study shows your java habit is actually good for you. From a lower stroke risk to fewer cavities, here are the best reasons to enjoy a cup or two.

"Coffee is incredibly rich in antioxidants, which are responsible for many of its health benefits," says Joy Bauer, RD, nutrition and health expert for Everyday Health and *The Today Show*. Its caffeine content may also play a protective role in some health conditions, but many of coffee's health perks hold up whether you go for decaf or regular.

According to this article, coffee can help avoid diabetes, skin cancer, stress, cavities, Parkinson's disease, breast cancer, heart disease, and head and neck cancers. Parkinson's disease runs in the family. That's another reason I'm so happy to have found this article.

It Hurts, But Just a Little

9/24/12 Are you watching out for your health? It's been pretty busy over here with Bear's retirement, the impending death of a loved one, Nima's visit from New York to say goodbye to her, and life in general. That might explain why I just plain forgot about watching out for mine – specifically, the pain in my shoulder.

Bear is officially retired, Nima's gone home, there's nothing more to do for Cheryl and it's life as usual so the pain is back. It hurts, but just a little. NSAIDS are out of the question, or are they?

I forgot to mention my computer is fried {Do you think I use it too much?}, so I pulled out my trusty laptop to write this blog... and found some interesting – if older – articles I'd saved. The first one to hit my eye {Figuratively, literally would have prompted a whole new discussion of painkillers!} was about the NSAID controversy. NSAID means Non-Steroidal Anti-Inflammatory Drug. Steroids have an adverse effect on the kidneys in that they strain the kidneys during filtration.

One of these articles discusses weighing the risk against the benefits of taking NSAIDS. I also have osteo-arthritis, but prefer to take Limbrel – a food medica-tion {By prescription only} to deal with the pain prevent-atively. I am afraid of damaging my kidneys further and am not willing to take NSAIDS. I went off the Limbrel for a while since it's so expensive, but noticed the pain in my elbows right away. That's when I decided the cost of the Limbrel was worth it if it meant no NSAIDS. That was my personal version of weighing the risks against the benefits.

Reading MedScape's coverage of the same study made me realize that 96% of the mild CKD patients in the study were unaware of their diagnose. This article also mentions that as of the 2011 date of publication far more patients were aware of their diagnose than during the actual study which took place between 1999 and 2004. I think it's this careful communication between nephrologist and patient that allows us, as the patients, to make informed decisions for ourselves.

I would like to see more of this, though. I'm still waiting for my own nephrologist to call me back about the steroidal drugs I was given during my cataract surgery although I clearly explained to the ophthalmologist that I have CKD and wanted nothing that would harm the kidneys. I'm beginning to wonder if doctors other than nephrologists know what drugs are harmful to the kidneys.

Fat Day

10/1/12   I feel fat and frustrated because I know what to do to lose weight, do it and still gain. It got so that I started to wonder if exercise were worth it. And counting calories? That went out the window. I never did get to the point of abandoning the renal diet, though. That's become sacrosanct, the way I wish losing weight was.

Following my usual method when I have a problem, I started researching. I remembered blogging about brown fat cells, but these were only recently discovered and no one knows how to access them yet. In case you forgot, brown fat cells gobble up other fat cells or something like that. I'd have to revisit the blog about them to be more specific, but I fear if I leave this page it will disappear. This is all so new to me.

EurekAlert's article about long term weight loss after menopause gave me pause {I couldn't resist. I think I'm feeling better already}. Obviously I've been through menopause, but not so obviously had no idea that because of that my resting metabolism has decreased, so has my losing weight and keeping it off ability despite having no sugary drinks, fried food or desserts. Well, drastically cutting down on desserts. It helps that I know I'm lactose intolerant, but I certainly am having trouble working gluten sensitivity into my renal diet.

That wasn't enough for me though. I wanted to feel that I was like everyone else so I searched some more. I should mention here that belly fat holds a great deal of my excess weight or, at least it looks that way to me.

Why MNT's article "Belly Fat Increases Risk Of Death Even In People Of Normal Weight" should be comforting is beyond me, but it was and actually lessened my frustration a bit. The article cites a Mayo Clinic study in which it was suggested, "...that people of average weight who have extra fat in their stomach ave a higher risk of dying than obese people."

Am I interpreting this to mean it's better to be obese? I sure hope that is not the case. A few things became clear while writing this blog. I am trying to combine the renal diet with those for high cholesterol, lactose intolerance, and gluten sensitivity. I am not succeeding. My failure here is probably the cause of my weight gain so I'll see my renal nutritionist for help, keep on exercising , and go right back to counting calories. Problem solved.

Blue Monday – But Only When It Comes To Sugar

10/8/12   I take the blood tests quarterly because I was prescribed Pravastatin which might have an effect on the liver. Pravastatin is used with hyperlipidemia {High cholesterol}. Luckily for me, I have had no side effects from this drug. As with every other patient taking the drug, it wasn't even prescribed until after we had tried dietary changes, exercise and weight reduction. My body seems to have a mind of its own {Like the juxtaposition of body and mind?}, and paid no attention to any of my efforts; hence, the drug regimen.

It seems my A1C, a blood test which measures how your body handles sugar over a three month period, had risen again. This has been on a very slow incline for quite a while. Now it's 6.3. At 6.4, I officially have type 2 diabetes.

What is that specifically? Type 2 is the type that can be controlled by – surprise! – lifestyle changes, while type 1 is insulin dependent or the kind that requires a daily injection. But wait a minute! I already limit the sweets {Sugar} and make it a point to exercise, so how could this be?

When I asked my primary care physician to help me with this, she was able to print out material about diabetic exchanges for meals. I also made an appointment with my nutritionist so she could help me combine the renal, hyperlipidemia, diabetic, and hypertension diets I need to follow. But that's later on this month. Meanwhile, let's deal with the material I was given.

Lo and behold, sweets are only one aspect of the diet. I hadn't realized carbohydrates had so much to do with diabetes. It seems they turn into sugar. Now that I know this, it makes perfect sense. I just never made the connection. I learned that too many carbohydrates at the same time raise the blood sugar.

Well, I got myself another eye opener as I read. I always thought of carbohydrates as starches – bread, cereal, starchy vegetables, and the beans that I can't eat anyway since they're not on the renal diet. But I learned they are also milk and yoghurt {I have never been so thankful to be lactose intolerant}, and fruit. I wasn't terribly upset since I'm already limited to six units of starches, three of vegetables - starchy or not, three of fruit and one of dairy. Uh-oh, doesn't that mean I was already being careful about my food intake? What else was I going to have to struggle with?

It turns out the limit for each of the categories of food in the diabetic diet is more liberal than those on the renal diet. For example, Sunday morning I make gluten free, organic blueberry pancakes. They're simple, quick and tasty. Bear uses butter and syrup, but I like them plain. According to the diabetes exchange, one of these counts as a starch {1 4-inch pancake about ¼" thick} and ½ of a fruit exchange {One-half cup of canned or fresh fruit}. Wait, there's more. I used 1 teaspoon of extra virgin olive oil which is a fat exchange. Hmmmm, this is simply not that different from counting units for the renal diet.

Ah, so the diabetic exchange meal is not that much of a problem for me, it's combining the restrictions of the four diets I need to follow. I've already decided to follow the lowest allowable amount of anything. For instance, the diabetic exchange allows 2,300 mg. of sodium per day while the renal diet only allows 2,000 mg. I stay well under 2,000 mg.

I'm beginning to see that I can figure out how to do this myself, but I am so glad to have my nutritionist to verify my conclusions. You know, the government pays for your nutritionist consultation once a year - twice if you're on Medicare - if you have Chronic Kidney Disease. It's not a bad idea to make an appointment. You may surprise yourself by not being aware of new dietary findings about the renal diet or discovering you've accidentally fallen into some bad dietary habit.

Also, as expected, exercise is also important if you have diabetes. It helps keep your blood sugar levels under control. The recommendation is 30 minutes five times a week. I'm already striving for 30 minutes a day every day and don't want to let that go.

This One's For Cheryl... and Amy...and...

10/15/12 It's true, the world is a sadder place these days. Two dynamic women have lost their lives to cancer this week, and both of them touched me. One fought valiantly until there was nothing more to fight with. One didn't. The end result is they're both gone. The cause of their deaths? Cancer.

I simply accepted that Cheryl Cook Vincent and I would grow to be outrageous old ladies together. Now my partner in crime is no more and I am so sad. I cannot think of a single purpose her death served.

Or maybe I can. Let's take a little detour from the usual CKD related material and talk about cancer. It's my way of honoring both Cheryl and my cousin, Amy Bernard-Herman. Cancer is defined by the World English Dictionary as:

any type of malignant growth or tumour, caused by abnormal and uncontrolled cell division: it may spread through the lymphatic system or blood stream to other parts of the body.

One of these women went to her doctors regularly; the other hadn't been in decades. Had she gone, she would have been told pretty much the same as the one who did. Cancer is treatable in the early stages, sometimes even curable as with skin cancer, the most common form of cancer. Sometimes, it is not - as with some breast cancer which is the second leading cause of cancer deaths in women. For men, the second leading cause of cancer is prostate cancer.

It seems that cancer really covers over one hundred different diseases rather than just being a disease all by itself according to MedicineNet.com. Even though it may appear in different parts of the body once it's metastasized {Spread}, it's referred to by the site where the tumors first appeared.

For example, back in 1988, my father died of pancreatic cancer. The cancer had metastasized throughout his body by the time he died, but it was still referred to as pancreatic cancer.

Colon cancer caused Cheryl's death, directly or not. ow could she have known she had this disease? According to the Mayo Clinic, these are the symptoms {Although the disease may be asymptomatic in the early stages in which case a colonoscopy would have detected it}:

- A change in your bowel habits, including diarrhea or constipation or a change in the consistency of your stool
- Unexplained weight loss
- Rectal bleeding or blood in your stool
- Persistent abdominal discomfort, such as cramps, gas or pain
- A feeling that your bowel doesn't empty completely
- Weakness or fatigue

You may need a reminder as to just what these parts of the body are. According to WebMD, the colon is the last part of the digestive system. This is where fluid, salt, and some nutrients are removed from your body's wastes as the digestive process occurs. Peristalsis, or the movement of the muscles lining the colon, helps with this. The rectum is the last four inches of the colon, ending with the anus.

Cancer has stages just as CKD does. MedicineNet has a better explanation of just what this is and why it's done than I could have come up with.

The stage of a cancer is a measure of the extent to which a cancer has spread in the body. Staging involves evaluation of a cancer's size and its penetration into surrounding tissue as well as the presence or absence of metastases in the lymph nodes or other organs.

Staging is important for determining how a particular cancer should be treated… cancer therapies are geared toward specific stages. Staging of a cancer also is critical in estimating the prognosis of a given patient, with higher-stage cancers generally having a worse prognosis than lower-stage cancers.

Rest in peace Cheryl… and Amy… and every other person who has died of cancer.

No book news today, folks.

My Turn for a Biopsy

10/22/12   I went to my dermatologist – my skin specialist. That's something I do every five years or so. There are multiple instances of melanoma in my family history so I took it upon myself to undergo a full body scan at least that often.

According to the Merriam-Webster Dictionary of Medical Terms,

a melanoma is a benign or malignant skin tumor containing dark pigment.

The doctor usually finds some little skin tags that can be snipped off so they don't get in my way or some suspicious mole to be scrapped off so it doesn't turn into cancer later on. This time was a little different.

My dermatologist found a couple of lesions that looked suspicious to her and asked my permission to freeze them off. I never agreed to anything so quickly before. The procedure is called cryosurgery which my dermatologist's medical group defines as

the treatment of lesions with the application of a cold substance. In most cases, liquid nitrogen is used to destroy the lesion.

Cold vastly understates the actual feeling.

Lesion sounded like a dirty word to me so I looked it up. The second definition of the word on The Free Online Dictionary is

A localized pathological change in a bodily organ or tissue.

That helped. While blisters did form as my dermatologist warned me they might, the one on my face is dried up and gone while the one on my leg is in a slightly uncomfortable holding pattern after eight days. I've always believed in not sweating the small stuff and this is small stuff in comparison to what happened next.

You guessed it. One week after losing a family member to breast cancer, I had not one, but two, biopsies. Being an eternal optimist, I was not even thinking about the possibilities this could bring to mind until I got the results. I'm great at acting immediately when necessary but also great about waiting until there is a necessity instead of going off halfcocked.

This may be a little hard to believe but just as I was about to hit the publish button on the blog site, my internet went down. I immediately got a call from the dermatologist's office telling me the biopsy came back benign {Harmless}... and the internet came back up. Wow!

Referring to another of the dermatology practice's handouts, I confirmed my thinking that

A biopsy is the removal of a small sample of a growth on the skin by your dermatologist. The sample is then sent to a pathologist, a doctor who examines this sample under a microscope and renders a diagnosis regarding the type of growth of disease present.

The area was numbed so I could have watched the process if I'd cared to. I am a firm adherent to recent research findings that NOT watching a medical procedure lessens the patient's pain {None here} and anxiety {Well...}.

As usual, I had to know exactly what the procedure was, and without watching it. Medilexicon was really helpful here. They define the punch biopsy as

any method that removes a small cylindric specimen for biopsy by means of a special instrument that pierces the organ directly, or through the skin, or a small incision in the skin.

A punch biopsy was performed, and I've got the three stitches to prove it! The stitches don't bother me a bit since the pressure bandages protect them. Depending upon which source you check, pressure bandages are used to stop bleeding {If I bled, I didn't know about it} or to prevent fluid from accumulating in the wound. Unfortunately, the keloids {Extra scar tissue formed over a wound} from biopsies in the same area twenty years ago may now have keloids of their own.

I actually saw the 'plugs' that were removed from my breast. It's not something a doctor usually offers to show you, but since all my questions were answered as I asked them, I figured I'd ask to see the plugs. And they were shown to me.

Read, Read, Read

10/29/12 I'm a voracious reader. I read everything: in-structions, food labels, medicine bottles, research, fiction, non-fiction, and my doctors' notes. In ***What Is It and How Did I Get It? Early Stage Chronic Kidney Disease***, I wrote about keeping a file for yourself for each doctor you see.

I began requesting copies of my doctor visit reports as well as my blood and urine tests so I could have my own file at home and stay on top of whatever I needed to. With these copies, my home files would be much more thorough. I was feeling burned by my previous P.A.'s failure to pick up on the low readings for the estimated GFR and felt I had to be my own case manager. I still do and find both the nephrol-ogist and my primary care physician agree with me.

Not a single doctor that I've seen for a test or a consultation has ever refused or been difficult about making certain I receive these copies. Most {The one exception was a rheum-atologist I encountered after the book was published who not only charged for these copies, but had me doing the telephone run around just to request them.} have encour-aged me to keep my own, thorough medical files at home. I suspect it may have made life easier for these doctors, too, since there was no calling other doctors to fax reports or request-ing them from labs. I had them and could fax them over to whichever doctor needed to see them immediately.

I have been adding quite a bit to these files recently due to the cataract surgery, sleep apnea apparatus, allergies, biopsies, cryosurgery, and an asthma scare. I have been a bit of a medical mess lately. Ever notice that things happen in threes? I'm beginning to think they may happen in sixes. At any rate, I began to doubt my own advice until I read an article on Medpage Today.

Opening MDs' Notes to Patients Wins Support

Patients who viewed their doctors' notes reported feeling more in control of their care and practiced better medication adherence, a study showed.

I have to agree that I do feel more in control when I read the doctors' notes. I'm also something of an over-achiever, so I want to see my success at whatever was instructed – provided I understand it and agree with it – reflected in my doctors' notes.

As for my doctors writing more clear and easily understood notes once they realized I would be reading them, well.... maybe it's because they know I'm going to research that mine don't do this. Wait a minute; I used to spend quite a bit of time researching. It seems to me that I spend less and less time these days, but am not certain if that's due to the growth of my knowledge base or if doctors really are writing in a way their patients can understand.

The other article that caught my eye was this one from EurekAlert.org.

Medication beliefs strongly affect individuals' management of chronic diseases, MU expert says

Health practitioners should use behavior-change tactics so patients take medications as prescribed

Nearly half of patients taking medications for chronic conditions do not strictly follow their prescribed medication regimens. Failure to use medications as directed increases patients' risk for side effects, hospitalizations, reduced quality of life and shortened lifespans. Now, a University of Missouri gerontological nursing expert says patients' poor adherence to prescribed medication regi-mens is connected to their beliefs about the necessity of prescriptions and concerns about long-term effects and dependency.

I readily accept that your beliefs dictate your behavior. For example, my PCP was worried that I might be developing asthma and prescribed a steroid inhaler plus a daily allergy pill until I could see my immun-ologist. She was being cautious, but the QVAR could cause oral thrush – a fungal condition – if I didn't rinse my mouth and teeth carefully enough. That was scary. A medication that could cause another condition? Hmmmm, it did allow me to breathe freely, though. After a couple of weeks, I became even more uncom-fortable since I believed I was developing a depend-ence on the QVAR. For once in my life, I didn't re-search that. I just stopped taking it. When I did get to see my immunologist, I suggested stress might be causing the ferocious cough and the difficulty catching my breath afterward. Not only did I have all these annoying medical problems I mentioned above, but my good buddy and my cousin died in the same week. It was a rough patch in my life unlike any I'd exper-ienced in the last twenty years.

My immunologist listened to me and suggested breathing exercises that might help since I wasn't interested in any more pills or other medication. At my request, she wrote the instructions for yoga breathing in her notes. And, of course, gave me a copy.

As for the article's mention of mechanical reminders to take your medication, I still wouldn't take med-ication if I didn't agree with the purpose for taking it. I do think I should have been more responsible and spoken with my doctor before I just stopped, but who says I was thinking clearly.

Fruits, Vegetables, and Staten Island

11/5/12   I brought up my daughters on Staten Island which is still part of New York City. Staten Islanders often call themselves 'the forgotten borough.' Nima, my Staten Is-land daughter, and I talked last night about how the food that defrosted in the freezer dur-ing the no electricity time during Hurricane Sandy has refrozen now that the power is back on.

Sometimes, people don't realize that defrosted frozen food must be tossed, not refrozen; it's no longer safe to eat. You can see {And smell} that most of the refrig-erator food is no longer edible after five days without electricity. I would-n't trust the rest of it. There's a reason we refrigerate food.

According to the United States Department of Agriculture's Food Safety and Inspection Service, these are guidelines to follow.

Always keep meat, poultry, fish, and eggs refrigerated at or below 40 °F and frozen food at or below 0 °F. This may be difficult when the power is out. {Or impossible with five days of no electricity even if you've kept the refrigerator and freezer doors closed. Please, take no chances.}

Keep the refrigerator and freezer doors closed as much as possible to maintain the cold temperature. The refrig-erator will keep food safely cold for about 4 hours if it is unopened. A full freezer will hold the temperature for ap-proximately 48 hours (24 hours if it is half full) if the door remains closed.

There's been new research that indicates fruits and vege-tables are more important to CKD patients than originally thought. Keep this in mind when you restock your refrig-erator.

This article appeared in The Kidney Group of South Florida's blog a few days ago. They originally located the article in HealthDay News. {San Diego hosted the American Society of Nephrology's annual meeting this past week-end, which was the source of quite a bit of new information.}

"After three years, consuming fruits and vege-tables or taking the oral medication reduced a marker of metabolic acidosis and preserved kidney function to similar extents. Our findings suggest that an apple a day keeps the neph-rologist away," study author Dr. Nimrit Goraya, of Texas A&M College of Medicine, said in a univer-sity news release.

Apparently, some CKD suffers have metabolic systems that are severely acidic. Fruits and vegetables are highly alkaline. This may counteract the acidity in the patients mentioned above AND those that have less metabolic acidosis (acid in the body).

What is not mentioned in the findings of the study is whether or not the CKD patients adhered to their fruit and vegetable restrictions. I am limited to three servings of each daily with their serving sizes limited according to the fruit or vegetable. For instance, I can consume three apricot halves during the same day, but only two peach halves,

I've written repeatedly about the prevalence of Chronic Kidney Disease. Now the public is beginning to understand. Consumer Reports, a magazine you should know if you've ever bought a car, an electronic device or anything else you need information about before buying now has a Chronic Kidney Disease Site.

From Veterans' Day Salt to Dense Breasts

11/12/12 Veterans' Day is observed today, although it was technically yesterday. People here in Arizona take their vet-erans seriously. For example, Texas Roadhouse offers the proverbial free lunch {Even though we all know these patriotic men and women have already paid the price.} for veterans.

As a Chronic Kidney Disease patient, I usually avoid this particular restaurant chain due to their heavy use of salt. I already knew they salted the French fries as they left the kitchen, so I simply ordered a Caesar Salad sans dressing and croutons as my side and ate very little of the full fat, full sodium Parmesan cheese topping my iceberg lettuce. The cheeseburger was a bit of a surprise. I rarely eat meat preferring ground turkey, which I buy 99% fat free. As for the cheese, they were perfectly willing to switch cheddar for the usual American. This was also full fat, full sodium but I wasn't concerned because I only planned to eat half of this 8 ounce burger, which meant only half the cheese, too.

What I hadn't figured on was the steak seasoning. I never use salt so when I took my first bite, it tasted as if I'd taken a bite out of some cow's errant salt lick. The waitress must have seen the look on my face. I didn't want to cause a fuss because the place was jam packed. Unbeknownst to me, the waitress told the manager who came over and insisted he make me a new burger with-out any seasoning. How kind of him... and I hadn't even mentioned that I have CKD.

So let's hear it for Texas Roadhouse for both their respect for veterans and the ease with which they accommodate food restrictions.

Keeping it salty today {Get it? Sodium? Salty?} Medicine-Net.com has an article about six top sources of sodium.

1. *Bread and rolls* - One piece of bread can have as much as 230 mg of sodium. That's 15% of the recommended daily amount. Although each serving may not sound like much, it can quickly add up throughout the day, with toast at breakfast, a sandwich at lunch, and a roll at dinner, etc.
2. *Cold cuts and cured meats* – Deli or pre-packaged turkey can have as much as 1,050 mg of sodium. It's added to most cooked and processed meats to reduce spoilage.
3. *Pizza* – One slice can have up to 760 mg of sodium. That means two slices accounts for a day's worth of salt.
4. *Poultry* – Packaged raw chicken often contains an added salt solution. Depending on how it's prepared the sodium level can quickly add up. Just 3 ounces of frozen and breaded chicken nuggets contains about 600 mg of sodium. {I have found no salt added poultry at Costco.}

5. *Soup* – This cold-weather staple can contain a day's worth of sodium in a single bowl. One cup of canned chicken soup can have up to 940 mg of sodium.
6. *Sandwiches* – Breads and cured meats are already high in salt, and putting them together with salty condiments like ketchup and mustard can add up to more than 1,500 mg of sodium in a single sandwich.

There was another surprise for me here. Chicken? I went through the material my nutritionist gave me and found that this did need to be limited since it was protein, but nothing about sodium. Notice #1 talks about 230 mg. of sodium being 15% of the recommend-ed daily amounts. It's a higher percentage for us. We are limited to 2,000 mg. of sodium daily – another 'perk' of having CKD – not the 2,400 mg. usually recommended. If you're following the teaspoon of salt guideline, it is 2,300 mg.

Take heart {Pun intended}, we are in good company. The American Heart Association made this recommendation on November 5th of this year.

"Americans of all ages, regardless of individual risk factors, can improve their heart health and reduce their risk of cardio-vascular disease by restricting their daily consumpt-ion of sodium to less than 1,500 mg," AHA chief executive officer Nancy Brown said in a statement.

A note about mammographies and dense breast tissue before we end. This article in *the New York Times* caught my eye because, even though I recently had biopsies due to lumps felt upon manual palpation, I also have dense breasts and was told so several years ago. Arizona has not passed this law yet. I was just lucky enough to have a caring mammographist.

In a move that has irked medical groups and delighted patient advocates, states have begun passing laws requiring clinics that perform mammograms to tell patients whether they have something that many women have never even heard of: dense breast tissue. Women who have dense tissue must, under those laws, also be told that it can hide tumors on a mammogram, that it may increase the risk of breast cancer and that they should ask their doctors if they need additional screening tests, like ultrasound or M.R.I. scans.

What's The Word I'm Looking For?

11/19/12   This is what I woke up.

Decreased kidney function leads to decreased cognitive functioning

Decreased kidney function is associated with decreased cognitive functioning in areas such as global cognitive abi-lity, abstract reasoning and verbal memory, according to a study led by Temple University. This is the first study des-cribing change in multiple domains of cognitive functioning in order to determine which specific abilities are most affected in individuals with impaired renal function.

EurekAlert! managed to blow whatever was left of my mind before I even had my morning coffee. {I do relish those two cups of this java joy a day.} I was stunned. I know I've been grasping for the right word when I speak and wondered why this was happening at the relatively young old age of 65. I'd accepted this would eventually happen, but later… you know, when I was old.

I started thinking about cognitive functioning and wondered what that really meant to me as a Chronic Kidney Disease patient. According to Mosby's Medical Dictionary, 8th edition, cognitive function is defined as

an intellectual process by which one becomes aware of, perceives, or comprehends ideas. It involves all aspects of perception, thinking, reasoning, and remembering.

Is that why I'm so slow to pick up the clues other people are dropping all around me? Is that why I have sudden revelations about a comment or an event days, sometimes weeks, after they occur? I have slowed down.

There is no question {Hah! I was about to write "in my mind," but that would be cognitive, wouldn't it?} of that. I see it in the way my lists have lists of their own. I see it in my preference for doing film where you only need to mem-orize a few scenes each day, instead of theatre where you need to have the entire script mem-orized before the play opens. And I see it in the way I have to carefully order – in writing – what I'd like the class to learn each day for my college work. I'll miss that off the cuff ability I seem to have lost.

But wait a minute, what is this "global cognitive ability"? Back to the dictionary. I couldn't find anything for global, but we know that means across the board or including all aspects so I didn't delve any further into that part of the phrase. The American Heritage Medical Dictionary tells us that cognitive ability is

The mental faculty of knowing, which includes perceiving, recognizing, conceiving, judging, reasoning, and imagining.

So we are slower at these skills since we have CKD. Add to that the slowing down we usually associate with age and we are slower yet. Well, no wonder I've noticed

I'm slowing down! I have two separate causes for that.
But here's the important part for me: I am simply
slowing down a bit. I am not stopping. I am not giving
up because it's taking a little longer to figure out what
it all means and what that word is I'm looking for.
There's an old writer's joke that is apt here.

Question: What is a synonym?
Answer: The word you use that means the
same as the one you wanted to use but forgot
how to spell.

It will get done, whatever it is. I'm actually
sort of comforted that there is a reason for
my lapses, my stopping to think a little harder.

Lest you start to become upset at this study's
findings, I'm including a quote from the study
which should set your mind at rest {Simply
cannot avoid using that word today.}.

"The brain and kidney are both organs that are
affected by the cardiovascular systems," said
the study's lead author, Adam Davey, associate
professor of public health in Temple's College
of Health Professions and Social Work. "They
are both affected by things like blood pressure
and hypertension, so it is natural to expect that
changes in one organ are going to be linked
with changes in another."

Bottom line: Everything affects everything, so
why worry? Follow your renal diet, exercise,
sleep and take any medications you need

to. Then have a good laugh {Preferably at your own expense.} and call me in the morning. The findings of the study don't change any-thing; they just help us understand.

Appy Trails to You

11/26/12   As any of my family members will tell you, I may not be the first around here to try something that's electronically new but I like exploring and am always de-lighted to find one app {Application} or another that makes my life easier.

For example, I've written several times about KidneyDiet, the app for counting electrolytes, fluids and calories. In ***What Is It and How Did I Get It? Early Stage Chronic Kidney Disease***, I wrote about carrying a pad and pen to keep track of these. Obvious-ly, that was before the app was developed. Now all I need is my phone… or iPad if I have it with me. I could always check it out on my laptop, too. The point is I'm not tied to my desktop to use the app.

Apparently, doctors have started to see the electronic light, too. According to the August 19, 2012, *NY Times*, apps may become part of your prescription and – get ready – be paid for by your insurance. I bought my KidneyDiet app this year and had intended to claim it on my taxes as a health cost, but to have my insurance pay for it? That's not only interesting; it's astounding at the moment. Of course, any new concept is. Here's to seeing this become part of our medical futures!

In addition to KidneyApp, I recently read about other apps. Being pre-diabetic, I was particularly interested in the one dealing with that disease. I thought it was another keeping-track-of-what-you-eat app. According to the article I men-tioned, it reads as if it's a doctor in your phone, or iPad, or laptop, or desktop. In other words, it does a lot more than track. This app, called DiabetesManager, does collect information about blood sugar levels, meds {Medication} and diet as we'd expect, but it can do so by wirelessly linking with the patient's glucose monitor.

One of the biggest reasons I don't use KidneyApp consistently is that information needs to be manually en-tered. I realize this is nothing more than laziness on my part but I'm human – glucose monitors are not. That also means no chance of human error in entering the information; say as in a finger slip so that the incorrect information is being entered.

I was still being amazed that such a thing could be done {Remember I'm 65. I didn't grow up with elect-ronics.} when I mentally blown out of the water by this statement:

DiabetesManager then gives advice to a patient, perhaps suggesting the best food after recording a low mid-day blood-sugar reading. It also uses an algorithm to analyze the medical data and send clinical recommendations to the doctor. WellDoc {That's the developer of Diabetes-Manager} says that in a clinical trial

DiabetesManager was shown to reduce signif-icantly the blood sugar levels in diabetes patients.

It gets even better. According to the company, as of August of this year, two unidentified insurance companies agreed to pay the hefty $100 per month cost of the app. Let me get this straight – diabetics get a doc in the pocket that insurance pays for? Sign me up! Oh wait, I don't have diabetes.

There are similar apps being developed for heart problems, too, as well as for physical therapy and rheumatoid arthritis. Maybe it has to do with my age, which means a history of personal doctor visits for information – then library research – on to internet research – and learning to track by hand, that I find this incredible. I know it's right here, but I keep think-ing it's the science fiction of my youth.

While the FDA has already approved DiabetesManager, it won't be available by prescription – yes, your doctor must prescribe it – before 2013.

Exercising My Options

12/3/12 According to a study published in *Diabetes Care* this past July: Weight control through diet and ex-ercise can prevent most cases of type 2 diabetes in American women over age 50...

I am a woman. I am an American. I am over the age of 50. And I have Chronic Kidney Disease which can be a cause of diabetes. Therefore, I am also confused.

Why, you ask? Easy, I've just finished reading an essay in *Physician*. In this essay, a point is made in the form of a question.

What if, believe it or not, when it comes to people with Type II diabetes, diet and exercise don't affect the incidence of heart attack, stroke, or hospital admission for angina or even the incidence of death?

Okay, so my wildest dream of not having to exercise to avoid illness has finally come true. Or has it? I looked over the articles I'd saved about my nemesis. It was a lot easier to force myself to exercise four years ago than it is now. My knees troubled me a bit then, but that was it. Now it's the knees, right hip, feet, and shoulders. I honestly do exercise, but it's not half as much fun as it used to be. Sure enough, in the articles I'd saved, I ran right into a bunch of reasons to keep up the exercise.

Statin therapy and physical fitness amounted to a one-two punch for lowering mortality risk in a large cohort of middle-age and older patients with dyslipidemia followed for 10 years.

Damn! I have dyslipidemia {High cholesterol} and periodically need to pay closer attention to it. According to this study originally printed in *The Lancet*, I need to keep exercising – if not to prevent myself from de-veloping the horrors of Type II Diabetes possible out-comes, then to keep the dyslipidemia under control… and I need to keep watching my diet.

Well, what about my knees and my other hurting parts that make me NOT want to exercise? The best quote I found came from Dr. Candice Johnstone at the Radio-logical Society of North America's press briefing this year when she spoke about exercising in moderation.

"I was not surprised by these results. This is more like common sense," added Johnstone, who is from the Medical College of Wisconsin in Milwaukee. "This adds to information people have to use to design their own exercise program."

Dr. Johnstone's reference to common sense seems like… well, common sense. If it hurts, don't do it. If you can do it with modification so that no pain is incurred, do it. You try not to poke at a tooth that hurts, don't you? So why poke at a joint that hurts?

All right now, just one more article. This one from the Centers for Disease Control and Prevention just a-bout convinced me I should be happy about exercis-ing.

Most weight loss occurs because of decreased caloric intake. However, evidence shows the only way to *maintain* weight loss is to be engaged in regular physical activity.

I can accept that. But what was the convincing part of the article is this:

Physical activity also helps to–
- Maintain weight.
- Reduce high blood pressure.
- Reduce risk for type 2 diabetes, heart attack, stroke, and several forms of cancer.
- Reduce arthritis pain and associated disability.
- Reduce risk for osteoporosis and falls.
- Reduce symptoms of depression and anxiety.

Now I remember why I started exercising. I love life. I love avoiding extra medication for ailments I could have handled with lifestyle changes. I love moving and feeling alive.

Back to the Salt Minds

12/10/12   Here we are right smack in the middle of Chanukah with Christmas and Kwanzaa coming up. We've read all the health articles about how to plan our party eating and we all know to avoid sodium since it causes so much havoc with blood pressure which causes further problems, right? Maybe not.

Be prepared to have your minds blown {Ahem, I am a child of the 60s.}.

Scant Evidence That Salt Raises BP, Review Finds

The evidence for health benefits associated with salt reduction is controversial and the "concealment of scientific uncertainty" is a mistake, researchers suggested.

So, what does this mean for us as Chronic Kidney Disease patients? Well... let's go back to CKD basics for
a moment. We are restricted as far as the three Ps {Protein, potassium, phosphorous} and sodium, not to mention fluid intake and – for some of us – caloric intake. {That's odd, these restrictions don't seem that complicated anymore, but when I type them, they look a bit daunting.}

Okay, so sodium. Too much sodium can lead to hypertension {Or can it?}, which may lead to CKD. You already have CKD. You are still at risk for edema, which is swell-

ing caused by fluid retention in the tissues of the
body. Since this is already a potential problem for CKD
pat-
ients, why exacerbate it?

This is what I wrote about sodium in *What Is It and
How Did I Get It? Early Stage Chronic Kidney Disease.*

What makes it worse is that there is no internal mechanism that tells us if we need more or less salt. CKD
sufferers are in a spot because the kidneys are the
only route by which to eliminate excess salt.

Basically, sodium balances fluid levels outside your
cells. You need it because it is responsible for
watering your cells. This watering is the prompt for
potassium to dump waste [cell process by-
products] from your cells. Sodium does deal with
other functions of the body, but this is a pretty
important one.

If you have damaged kidneys and cannot excrete most
of the sodium you ingest, you're up against higher
blood pressure {Is that still true?} which may
worsen your CKD which may further cut down on your
elimination of sod-ium and so on and so forth in an
ever spiraling cycle. In addition, for CKD patients, too
much sodium causes fluid retention, thereby causing
swelling, further resulting in weight gain, leading
to shortness of breath. That's why your nephrologist
asks if you've experienced shortness of breath.

It gets worse. This is also from *What Is It and How Did
I Get It? Early Stage Chronic Kidney Disease*.

Too much sodium can increase your need for potassium. While potassium is a necessity since it dumps waste from your cells, it also helps the kidneys, heart and muscles to function normally. Too much potassium can cause irreg-ular heart beat and even heart attack. This can be the most immediate danger of not limiting your potassium.

That is a simple, direct and universally accepted explan-ation of the horrors of sodium for CKD patients. But is it still true for you? With these newly uncovered con-troversies, who knows? Speak with your nephrologist, but use common sense, too. I would not recommend running for the salt shaker under any cir-cumstances, but is it safe to eat the fresh made potato chips you ordered at the local brewery {Not that I drank any beer. Oh – I mean, not that you drank any beer.} when you tasted a bit of salt on them?

I thought about handling my renal diet party by party and that has worked well for me. Prior to that, I had a forbid-den list I carried around in my head. That was a total bust. I would become frustrated at all the foods I couldn't eat even though they were beautifully and enticingly dis-played in front of me and just go whole hog. Then I had to deal with the guilt, to say nothing of the bodily discomfort that I felt after.

Yes, party by party is better for me. But that's not all. I am analytic, so I peruse the offerings and then – slowly – mentally check off what I can ingest, all the while socializing. That works for me. So does the old dieter's motto: do-not-stay-seated-at-the-table-with-that-wonderfully-aromatic-food-in-front-of-you.

Feeling well armed to go to your holiday parties with sodium intake well in hand? Go party!

The Flu Flew By

12/17/12   'Tis the season to be jolly… and get the flu. You'll be in crowds at your holiday parties, even in stores when you get your shopping done. Everyone's got to eat, even Scrooge, so you will be in the markets – and crowds – whether you want to be or not.

Uh-oh, so what do you do about the flu? According to Dec. 3, 2012's Medpage Today, the flu has arrived early this year. Bah! Humbug! Just in time for the holiday sea-son.

The flu season is officially under way about a month ear-lier than usual, the CDC announced on a call marking the beginning of National Influenza Vaccination Week. {For your information, that was Dec. 2-8 this year}

"This is the earliest regular flu season we've had in nearly a decade, since the 2003-2004 flu season," CDC director Thomas Frieden, MD, MPH, said on a confer-ence call with reporters.

Who even knew there was a National Influenza Vaccination Week? Reminder: as a Chronic Kidney Disease patient, you already have a compromised immune system. Help yourself to avoid the flu by getting that vaccine. In some cases {You'll have to ask your health-care worker if you are part of this group}, you may be able to take the nasal vaccine. This is especially helpful if you have a great dislike for injections, but if you can't because you have CKD, just look away during the shot. That has been proven to make it easier to handle the fear, as I wrote about in an earlier blog. By the way, Medicare covers the cost of the flu shot. So, again I ask what do you do about the flu? According to Healthfinder.gov, you can protect yourself from the flu by doing the following.

Getting the flu vaccine is the most important step in protecting yourself from the flu. Here are some other things you can do to keep from getting and spreading the flu.

- Stay away from people who are sick.
- If you are sick, stay home for at least 24 hours after your fever
- is gone.
- Wash your hands often with soap and warm water.
- Try not to touch your nose, mouth, or eyes.
- Cover your mouth and nose with a tissue when you cough or sneeze.

Most of this sounds fairly obvious. But there are people who simply sneeze and cough into the air around them. That got me to thinking. Do you find yourself shying away from certain people who do the same? Maybe you should.

Since the cataract surgery and the sealing off of my tear ducts, I am always touching my eyes to wipe away the extra moisture. Until I read this article, I'd always thought of myself as someone who doesn't keep touching my face. But that's not true, is it?

And how many people in this economy really do take off from work for 24 hours after their fevers break? Who can afford to do that? We have people struggling to hang on to minimum wage positions while a string of other people are ready and waiting for these same jobs.

It's worth thinking about this yourself. Remember when we were taught to cough or sneeze into the inside of our elbows? Looks like that's not as effective as stopping the particulate spray immediately at its source – your nostrils. Makes sense to me.

According to Rob Stein on NPR's Health News

"One big difference between this year and the 2003-2004 season is that so far the vaccine appears to be a very good match for the strains of flu that are circulating most wide-ly. That's important because one of the reasons officials are concerned is that one of the strains is similar to the 2003-2004 strain that caused so much illness and so many deaths."

I think that's good news. It sounds like good news. Is it good news? Why DID the 2003-2004 strain cause so much illness and so many deaths? Somehow, that's not as reassuring as I'd like it to be.

I wondered how to tell the difference between a cold and the flu. Since being diagnosed with CKD, I make it a point to take the flu vaccine annually, yet there have been times when I just didn't feel that well. I found my answer at ABC News.

"With influenza you might also feel very poorly, with aches and pains in your muscles and joints," said Dr. William Schaffner," chair of preventive medicine at Vanderbilt University Medical Center in Nashville, Tenn. "There's often a cough, too, which is much more prolonged and pronounced."

Renal Foodie

12/24/12   When I went to the market for the ingredients I needed for the dish I was to prepare for a family dinner, I became aware of just how carefully I look at nutrition labels {The number of people politely waiting for me to move out of the way and then aheming when I didn't notice them may have had something to do with that.} and wondered how many other people knew how to read them.

We are Chronic Kidney Disease patients. We do not have the luxury of tossing anything into our systems, yet we need to make the food we share with others tasty. How to do that?

DaVita has some holiday cooking tips of their own. Are you cooking a dish for a party and want to make sure it doesn't pack on the pounds? If you cook, use healthy recipe substitutions for your kidney diet dishes.

Listed are some ingredients a recipe may call for and the kidney-friendly substitute to use instead.

Recipe calls for:	Substitute with:
1 whole egg	2 egg whites or ¼ cup egg substitute
Sour cream or cream cheese	Low fat sour cream or low fat cream cheese
Sugar	Splenda® or other low

	calorie sweetener
Oil (for baking)	Unsweetened applesauce
Regular Jello®	Sugar-free Jello® or gelatin
Fruit packed in syrup	Fruit packed in juice

I do have to write something about the use of the sugar free products. I wouldn't use the substitutes, but would lower the amounts of sugar used in the recipe instead. Sugar is 15 calories per tablespoon and is much healthier than any substance that has been altered in any way. Until recently, I felt safe substituting un-sweetened applesauce for sugar, but with the recent pub-licizing of genetically modified foods, I don't trust the product anymore. I would expect to see some central clearing house to list GMOs in the near future.

According to Wikipedia Genetically modified foods (GM foods, or biotech foods) are foods derived from genet-ically modified organisms (GMOs), specifically, genetically modified crops. GMOs have had specific changes intro-duced into their DNA by genetic engineering techniques.

As I researched GMOs for this blog, it seemed to me art-icles were either written and posted by health proponents urging they be avoided or businesses promoting them. Craveat: this is not something I researched in depth and this is simply my opinion.

Good Bye to 2012 and Its Obesity

12/31/12   Today is the last day of 2012. That means you can start your new year's resolutions tomorrow. When you're done laughing, think about it. We make resolutions intending to keep them – at least I do – but something happens right about March something or other. We tend to forget what they are.

We could look at it another way. Pollyanna over here likes this way better. What has become part of your life as a former new year's resolution? For me, it's the renal diet and exercise. I actually feel bad when I can't exercise now. There's hope for me in the form of a possible cortisone injection to lubricate that hip that has eroded so much that it is bone on bone. I know you were really worried about that. {She wrote tongue in cheek.} Sometimes we need motivation to even think of resolutions. Jody Charnow provided that for me in the Dec. 26 issue of *Renal and Urology News*:

Overweight, Obesity Raise Kidney Disease Risk

A large study conducted in Thailand corroborates previous findings showing that overweight and obesity are assoc-iated with an increased likelihood of Chronic Kidney Disease (CKD). Subjects with CKD had a significantly higher mean BMI than those without CKD (25.36 vs. 24.04), as well as a significantly higher prevalence of abdominal obesity (35.7% vs. 25.3%). The investigators defined abdominal obesity as a waist circumference of 90 cm {That's 35 7/16 inches for the math challenged like me.} or greater for men and greater than 80 cm {This one is about 31 and a half inches.} for women.

Just in case you don't remember, BMI means Body Mass Index or a way of measuring the fat content of your body based on your height and weight. So why all the whining about not being able to exercise, you ask.

Read that article excerpt again. I already have Stage 3 Chronic Kidney Disease. How much worse do you think a lack of exercise – which leads to weight gain – is going to make my CKD? Technically {I just had to qualify that.}, I already am obese. I'm not that vain, but I want to stay at Stage 3 for the rest of my life and avoid dialysis completely. This is not the way to do it.

Let's try this another way – for those of you who can walk – untreated hypertension {High blood pressure} may also be one of the causes of CKD. According to the *New York Daily News*, exercise can lower your blood pressure. We already know that obesity is another possible cause of CKD. Here's the good part: while you're walking to lower your blood pressure, you're also exercising which means you're losing weight if you're consistent enough. Wow! Two for one here!

I found surprising information in that article. Who knew that fructose raises your blood pressure? The only time I'd heard it mentioned as a medical deficit is at the immunologist's. She had warned me that fructose should be avoided if you have allergies.

Potassium may also be a key in lowering your blood pressure. I've been draining my canned fruit and only occasionally having a fresh {Oh, all right, HALF a fresh} banana to control my potassium intake. Guess what. My blood pressure has gone up. Maybe I shouldn't be that surprised.

Oh no! The article also suggests losing weight. Looks like it always comes back to the same thing. A thinner body is a healthier body as long as we don't go past thinner to obscenely thin.

Until next year,
Keep living your life!

Index

A

B

C

D

E

F

G

H

Reviews for the former ***The Book of Blogs: Moderate Stage Chronic Kidney Disease, Part 1*** (Currently ***SlowItDownCKD 2011*** and ***SlowItDownCKD 2012***)

"If you have kidney disease, like I do, you can relate to what Gail Rae-Garwood has written here... very useful..."

"I got this when it was free, but have just now gotten around to browsing through it. These are the same blogs that I read and relied on for information as I went down the road of chronic kidney disease. If you need to know it, it's here or in part 2. I started with her book, ***What Is It and How Did I Get It?*** when I saw a flyer for it in my kidney doctor's waiting room. Much like Gail, I've been inhaling information about this issue, since I'm not one to sit around and trust someone to just tell me what to do. She has done her research. I have a few other books about kidney disease, but this one was the one that my husband likes the best when he was curious about my condition. The blogs cover most of this territory, but broken down in nice little blog type chapters. The only thing missing is a table of contents, but as I looked for the thing I wanted, I found I was re-reading things I'd forgotten about. So, browsing this volume and the second one as well can be helpful as a refresher course so to speak."

"This book is the only written resource I've found to answer the tough questions that come with Chronic Kidney Disease. Although our doctors are great at treating us, they aren't always available to give in depth answers or really explore the whys and hows of

a question. Rae-Garwood does an excellent job antici-
pating exactly the kinds of questions that came up for
us. Give it a try."

"I won a copy of this book when Gail had a contest. I
was happy to receive it to pass on to a family member
but skimmed it myself first. Since I read Gail's first
book and usually read her blogs I was familiar with
her style. Some of the posts I had read before but it's
all good info presented in a friendly, readable format.
I'm pretty sure that Gail has added an index to the
book which my copy does not have and that would be
a great addition. It seems like Gail has covered CKD
from every angle. I recommend this book for anyone
who has been diagnosed with CKD or knows someone
who has."

My Notes -

Have you read my other Chronic Kidney
Disease books?
available on Amazon.com and B&N.com
(print and digital)

What Is It and How Did I Get It?
Early Stage Chronic Kidney Disease
SlowItDownCKD 2011
SlowItDownCKD 2013
SlowItDownCKD 2014
SlowItDownCKD 2015
SlowItDownCKD 2016

Follow the blog at
https://gailraegarwood.wordpress.com

SLOWITDOWNCKD
EARLY AND MODERATE STAGE CHRONIC KIDNEY DISEASE

On Instagram, Pinterest, and Twitter go to
@SlowItDownCKD

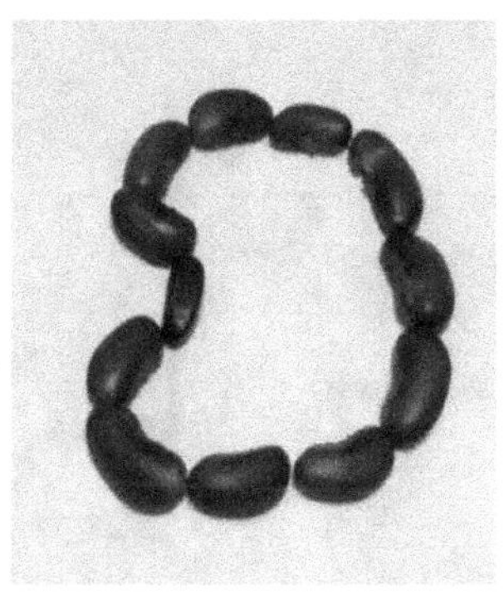

And then, there's the Facebook page at
**https://www.facebook.com/
SlowItDownCKD/**

Don't forget you can email me at
SlowItDownCKD@gmail.com

**If you'd like to read a time travel romance
(available on Amazon.com
in both digital and print)**

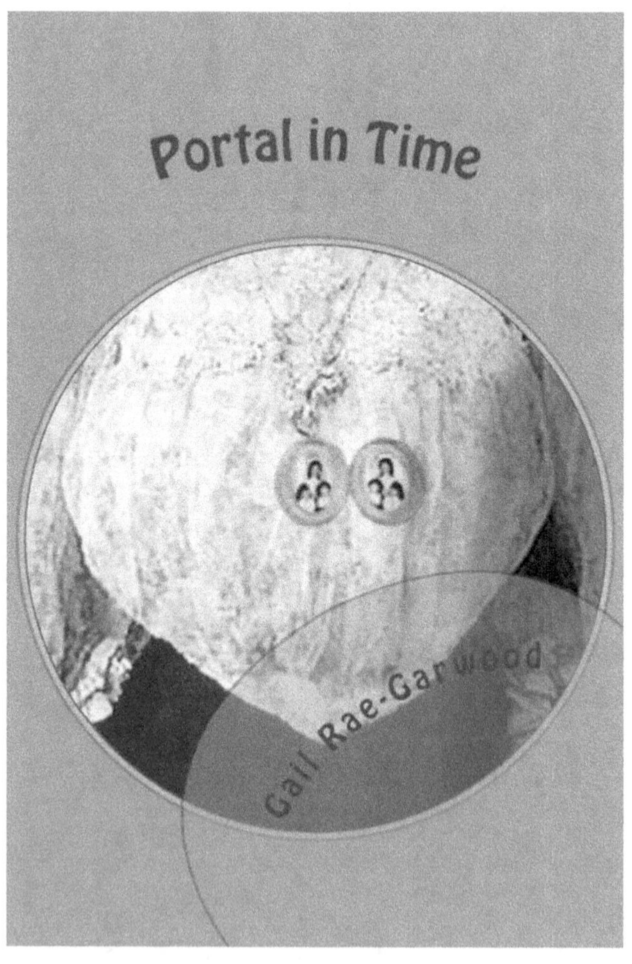